Assessing the United States Institute of Peace Jennings Randolph Senior Fellowship

Committee to Review the United States Institute of Peace Senior Fellows Program

Development, Security, and Cooperation
Policy and Global Affairs

NATIONAL RESEARCH COUNCIL
OF THE NATIONAL ACADEMIES

THE NATIONAL ACADEMIES PRESS
Washington, D.C.
www.nap.edu

THE NATIONAL ACADEMIES PRESS 500 Fifth Street, N.W. Washington, D.C. 20001

NOTICE: The project that is the subject of this report was approved by the Governing Board of the National Research Council, whose members are drawn from the councils of the National Academy of Sciences, the National Academy of Engineering, and the Institute of Medicine. The members of the committee responsible for the report were chosen for their special competences and with regard for appropriate balance.

This project was supported by the United States Institute of Peace. Any opinions, findings, conclusions, or recommendations expressed in this publication are those of the author(s) and do not necessarily reflect the views of the organizations or agencies that provided support for the project.

International Standard Book Number 13:978-0-309-13014-1
International Standard Book Number 10:0-309-13014-X

Additional copies of this report are available from the National Academies Press, 500 Fifth Street, N.W., Lockbox 285, Washington, D.C. 20055; (800) 624-6242 or (202) 334-3313 (in the Washington metropolitan area); Internet, http://www.nap.edu.

Suggested citation: National Research Council. 2008. Assessing the United States Institute of Peace Jennings Randolph Senior Fellowship. Washington, D.C.: The National Academies Press.

Copyright 2008 by the National Academy of Sciences. All rights reserved.

Printed in the United States of America

THE NATIONAL ACADEMIES
Advisers to the Nation on Science, Engineering, and Medicine

The **National Academy of Sciences** is a private, nonprofit, self-perpetuating society of distinguished scholars engaged in scientific and engineering research, dedicated to the furtherance of science and technology and to their use for the general welfare. Upon the authority of the charter granted to it by the Congress in 1863, the Academy has a mandate that requires it to advise the federal government on scientific and technical matters. Dr. Ralph J. Cicerone is president of the National Academy of Sciences.

The **National Academy of Engineering** was established in 1964, under the charter of the National Academy of Sciences, as a parallel organization of outstanding engineers. It is autonomous in its administration and in the selection of its members, sharing with the National Academy of Sciences the responsibility for advising the federal government. The National Academy of Engineering also sponsors engineering programs aimed at meeting national needs, encourages education and research, and recognizes the superior achievements of engineers. Dr. Charles M. Vest is president of the National Academy of Engineering.

The **Institute of Medicine** was established in 1970 by the National Academy of Sciences to secure the services of eminent members of appropriate professions in the examination of policy matters pertaining to the health of the public. The Institute acts under the responsibility given to the National Academy of Sciences by its congressional charter to be an adviser to the federal government and, upon its own initiative, to identify issues of medical care, research, and education. Dr. Harvey V. Fineberg is president of the Institute of Medicine.

The **National Research Council** was organized by the National Academy of Sciences in 1916 to associate the broad community of science and technology with the Academy's purposes of furthering knowledge and advising the federal government. Functioning in accordance with general policies determined by the Academy, the Council has become the principal operating agency of both the National Academy of Sciences and the National Academy of Engineering in providing services to the government, the public, and the scientific and engineering communities. The Council is administered jointly by both Academies and the Institute of Medicine. Dr. Ralph J. Cicerone and Dr. Charles M. Vest are chair and vice chair, respectively, of the National Research Council.

www.national-academies.org

Committee to Review the United States Institute of Peace Senior Fellows Program

Major General William F. Burns (USA, retired), *Chair*, Carlisle, PA.

Burt S. Barnow, Associate Director for Research and Principal Research Scientist, Institute for Policy Studies, Johns Hopkins University, Baltimore, MD.

Joyce Davis, Senior Vice President, WITF, Inc., Harrisburg, PA.

P. Terrence Hopmann, Professor of International Relations and Director of the Conflict Management Program, The Paul H. Nitze School of Advanced International Studies (SAIS), Johns Hopkins University, Washington, DC; Professor Emeritus of Political Science, Brown University, Providence, RI.

Kathryn E. Newcomer, Professor and Associate Director, Trachtenberg School of Public Policy and Public Administration, George Washington University, Washington, DC.

Johanna Mendelson Forman, Senior Associate, Center for Strategic and International Studies, Washington, DC.

Karin von Hippel, Co-Director, Post-Conflict Reconstruction Project, and Senior Fellow, International Security Program, Center for Strategic and International Studies, Washington, DC.

Christine Wing, Senior Fellow and Project Coordinator, Strengthening Multilateral Approaches to Nuclear and Biological Weapons, Center on International Cooperation, New York University, New York, NY.

I. William Zartman, Jacob Blaustein Professor of International Organizations and Conflict Resolution, The Paul H. Nitze School of Advanced International Studies (SAIS), Johns Hopkins University, Washington, DC.

Staff

Jo Husbands, Ph.D., Senior Project Director
John Sislin, Ph.D., Study Director

PREFACE AND ACKNOWLEDGMENTS

Beginning in 1987, the United States Institute of Peace Jennings Randolph Senior Fellowship Program has brought just over 250 academics, practitioners, diplomats, and other individuals to Washington, DC, for ten-month residencies. The accomplishments of this group of experts over the past two decades have contributed directly to a better understanding and further analysis of the contributions of negotiations, conflict resolution measures, and specific policies such as arms control and humanitarian assistance to establishing and maintaining peace in volatile regions of the world. The authors of this report are pleased to contribute further to this effort through an evaluation of the program.

This report has been reviewed in draft form by individuals chosen for their diverse perspectives and technical expertise, in accordance with procedures approved by the National Academies' Report Review Committee. The purpose of this independent review is to provide candid and critical comments that will assist the institution in making its published report as sound as possible and to ensure that the report meets institutional standards for objectivity, evidence, and responsiveness to the study charge. The review comments and draft manuscript remain confidential to protect the integrity of the process.

We wish to thank the following individuals for their review of this report: Harley Balzer, Georgetown University; Sheila Buckley, Independent Consultant; Hrach Gregorian, Institute of World Affairs; Virginia Haufler, University of Maryland; Bruce Jentleson, Duke University; Robert Litwak, Woodrow Wilson International Center for Scholars; and George Lopez, University of Notre Dame.

Although the reviewers listed above have provided many constructive comments and suggestions, they were not asked to endorse the conclusions or recommendations, nor did they see the final draft of the report before its release. The review of this report was overseen by Lawrence Brown, University of Pennsylvania. Appointed by the National Academies, he was responsible for making certain that an independent examination of this report was carried out in accordance with institutional procedures and that all review comments were carefully considered. Responsibility for the final content of this report rests entirely with the authoring committee and the institution.

The committee wants to thank the members of the National Research Council staff who provided extensive input during the project. John Sislin, the study director, collected data, including fielding the surveys, and provided the analyses that went into this report. Jim Voytuk provided survey software. Jo Husbands participated in the design of the project and provided comments throughout the process. The committee is also grateful to staff at the United States Institute of Peace who provided data on Fellows and applicants alike. Finally, the committee is especially grateful to those former Fellows who participated in the study by completing the Fellows' survey, as well as those individuals who filled out the peace and security experts' survey. Although filling out surveys is tedious and often unrewarding, the committee hopes that the completion of this report will be valuable to the United States Institute of Peace in its continuing mission to increase knowledge on peace and security topics, as well as to others involved in senior fellowship programs such as this one.

Major General William F. Burns (USA, ret.), Chair

Contents

Preface and Acknowledgments		v
Summary		1
1	Overview	7
2	Characteristics of Applicants, Fellows, and Research Topics	19
3	Views of Former Fellows	35
4	Perceptions of the Peace and Security Community	61
5	Recommendations for the Next Step	71
Bibliography		77

Appendixes

A. Committee Members Biographical Information	78
B. Survey of Former Fellows	82
C. Survey of Peace and Security Experts	87
D. Top Foreign Policy Problems Identified by Chicago Council on Foreign Relations Interviews with Foreign Policy Leaders, 1986–2002	93

List of Tables and Figures

TABLES

TABLE 1-1 Summary of research questions, sources of information, and data collection techniques, 12

TABLE 1-2 Data from USIP, 13

TABLE 1-3 Number of Fellowships and number contacted by year of Fellowship, 15

TABLE 2-1 Type of employment of Fellows, 1987–2007, and applicants, 1997–2007, 24

TABLE 2-2 Types of research foci, 25

TABLE 2-3 Applicant research focus, 1997–2007, 26

TABLE 2-4 Applicant research focus by topic, 27

TABLE 2-5 Research topics of Fellows, 1987–2007, 28

TABLE 2-6 Research topics of Fellows by topic area, 29

TABLE 2-7 Geographic areas of focus, 29

TABLE 2-8 Geographic focus of applicants' proposed research by year, 30

TABLE 2-9 Geographic focus of applicants' proposed research by percentage, 31

TABLE 2-10 Geographic focus of Fellows' research by year, 32

TABLE 2-11 Geographic focus of Fellows' research by percentage, 33

TABLE 3-1 Distribution of respondents by year of Fellowship, 35

TABLE 3-2 Percentage of respondents reporting professional or career development activities by year of Fellowship, 37

TABLE 3-3 Percentage of Fellows engaging in various measures of productivity by year of Fellowship, 39

TABLE 3-4 Percentage of Fellows engaging in various activities by year of Fellowship, 40

TABLE 3-5 Respondents' perception of the overall quality of the Fellowship Program by period of Fellowship, 41

TABLE 3-6 Degree, by year of Fellowship, to which Fellows' expectations regarding mentoring or advising were met, 42

TABLE 3-7 Percentage of respondents, by period of Fellowship, who agreed that the Fellowship was useful in increasing network of colleagues, 44

TABLE 3-8 Major themes and examples of respondents' views of best and worst features of the Fellowship, 47

TABLE 3-9 Fellows' post-Fellowship activities by year of Fellowship, 51

TABLE 3-10 Percentage of respondents, by period of Fellowship, who agreed with various statements about the Fellowship, 53

TABLE 3-11 Whether respondents would recommend the Fellowship to others, 57

TABLE 3-12 Whether respondents have recommended the Fellowship to others, 57

TABLE 4-1 Familiarity with various senior peace and security fellowships, 63

TABLE 4-2 Mean familiarity with various senior peace and security fellowships, 64

TABLE 4-3 Prestige of various senior peace and security fellowships, 65

TABLE 4-4 Weighted prestige of various senior peace and security fellowships, 66

TABLE 4-5 Percentage of respondents who knew any USIP Jennings Randolph Senior Fellows, 66

TABLE 4-6 Respondents' views on importance of the Fellowships, 67

TABLE 4-7 Respondents' views on Fellows' output, 67

TABLE 4-8 Respondents' views on return on investment of the program, 68

TABLE 4-9 Whether respondent has ever recommended to anyone that s/he should apply for the Fellowship, 68

TABLE 4-10 Relationship between familiarity and recommendation by respondent, 69

TABLE 5-1 Top 5 foreign policy problems identified in Chicago Council on Foreign Relations interviews with foreign policy leaders, 1986–2002, 73

FIGURES

FIGURE 2-1 Number of Senior Fellowships awarded, 1987–2007, 19

FIGURE 2-2 Number of applicants, 1997–2007, 20

FIGURE 2-3 Ratio of number of Fellowships to applicants, 1997–2007, 21

FIGURE 2-4 Percentage of female Fellows, 1987–2007, and applicants, 1997–2007, 22

FIGURE 2-5. Percentage of Fellows, 1987–2007, and applicants, 1997–2007, who were U.S. citizens, 23

FIGURE 3-1 Percentage of respondents reporting professional or career development activities, 36

FIGURE 3-2 Percentage of respondents reporting engagement in activities by type, 38

FIGURE 3-3 Respondents' perception of the overall quality of the Fellowship program, 40

FIGURE 3-4 Degree to which Fellowship met Fellows' expectations by program aspect, 42

FIGURE 3-5 Degree of usefulness of Fellowship for Fellow by aspect, 43

FIGURE 3-6 Extent of opportunity to interact with various networks, 44

FIGURE 3-7 Percentage of respondents who agreed that ten months is the right duration for the Fellowship, 45

FIGURE 3-8 Post-Fellowship activities, 50

FIGURE 3-9 Percentage of respondents who agreed with various statements about the Fellowship, 52

FIGURE 3-10 Percentage of respondents' saying the Fellowship was helpful in various ways, 54

FIGURE 3-11 Changes to respondents' networks by type of actor, 55

FIGURE 3-12 Respondents' degree of satisfaction with various characteristics of the Fellowship, 56

BOX 4-1 Descriptions of Senior Fellowships Programs, 62

Summary

The United States Institute of Peace (USIP) is an independent, nonpartisan, national institution established and funded by the U.S. Congress. The goals of the USIP are to help prevent and resolve violent international conflicts; promote post-conflict stability and development; and to increase conflict management capacity, tools, and intellectual capital worldwide. One way the USIP meets those goals is through the Jennings Randolph Program for International Peace, which awards Senior Fellowships to outstanding scholars, policymakers, journalists, and other professionals from around the world to conduct research at the USIP. The Fellowship Program began in 1987, and 253 Fellowships have been awarded through 2007.

This report presents a preliminary assessment of the Fellowship Program. The committee's charge was to address the following questions:
1. What are the characteristics of USIP Senior Fellows and how have those characteristics changed over time?
2. What issues do Fellows research and how do those issues relate to the mandate of the USIP and to U.S. foreign policy?
3. How do former Fellows and members of the external peace and security community perceive the program with respect to its:
    a. Impact on the Senior Fellows themselves;
    b. Advancement of the mandate of the USIP; and
    c. Contribution to increased knowledge or awareness of peace and security issues?

The committee collected information on the Fellowship Program from three primary sources: data collected on applicants and Fellows by the USIP, a survey of former Fellows, and a survey of experts in the broader peace and security community. With this information, the committee was able to directly address the first task above. The committee's ability to respond to the second task was limited. This was partly due to an absence of data and partly to reduced access to USIP experts. In response to the third task, the committee began to survey external experts. Although the survey was limited, it raises several interesting findings. The committee's findings are based on the data collected for this study in order to address the charge. The committee believes that the report addresses the issues raised in its charge to the level that the resources available permitted.

Key findings were divided into three categories, roughly parallel to the three questions in the committee's charge. Regarding the first task, and to a lesser extent the second, the data showed that:

- Each year, USIP selects between 7 and 16 percent (mean of 11 percent) of applicants to become Fellows.
- Most Fellows and applicants are male and academics. Seventeen percent of Fellows are female (where gender is known). On average, 45 percent were U.S. citizens.
- Overall, conflict prevention, management, and resolution were the most common topics for Fellow's research, followed by conflict, political systems, and international organization and law topics.

- In terms of geographical focus, many Fellows' work fit into the "global" category. Focus on Eastern Europe and the Former Soviet Union seemed to peak from 1994 to 2000. The Middle East and North Africa foci were popular from 1997 to 2001, and from 2003 to 2007 (in particular most of the 2007 Fellows were working on this region). Research on sub-Saharan Africa ranked fourth among the areas of geographic focus for Fellows' research

Additional data and further information about these trends over time are presented in Chapter 2.

Regarding the third task, and based on the survey of Fellows:

- A challenge for monitoring and evaluation is that a number of Fellows could not be located.
- Fellows gave the program high marks.
- Fellows are very active in conducting research and disseminating information to multiple stakeholders. USIP receives substantial benefit from the Fellows' residencies in Washington, DC.
- Fellows have many opportunities to network with others and are generally satisfied with the amount of opportunities.
- Fellows tend to remain in contact with USIP and participate in USIP activities after the Fellowship ends.
- Most Fellows reported ten months to be an appropriate duration for the Fellowship, although some thought that the Fellowship should be longer.
- Finally, Fellows are not certain how well known the Fellowship is, though they think the Fellowship is prestigious.

Finally, regarding the third task and to a lesser extent, the second, the preliminary survey of experts found:

- A wide majority of respondents (79 percent) had some familiarity with the USIP Fellowship Program. More than two-thirds of respondents knew one or more fellows.
- External commentators gave the Fellowship relatively high marks for prestige. Forty-three percent of respondents rated the program at least a 4 on a scale of 1 to 5.
- Respondents reported that the Fellowship was seen to be more important by the experts as a networking opportunity and a means to increase knowledge. There was less agreement on its importance in developing new tools to respond to conflict.
- The Fellows' role was seen by respondents as somewhat more important in supporting policymakers by providing information than in performing cutting edge research.
- Finally, while respondents were familiar with the program and many knew a Fellow, a majority had not recommended to anyone that s/he apply for the Fellowship.

Since this is the first, formal evaluation of the Fellowship Program, the committee placed significant emphasis on providing advice to USIP in the form of recommendations—for next steps to remove the limitations on information about some aspects of the Fellowship and to advance monitoring and evaluation by the USIP. The recommendations are contained in the final chapter of the report, along with more detailed information about the some of the recommendations as well as supporting material where further explanation may help to clarify the committee's proposals.

Gathering Additional Data

USIP has accumulated a substantial amount of information about applicants and Fellows, but the committee also encountered some significant limitations. The spreadsheet created by USIP (data categories are presented in Table 1-2) is a useful tool for collecting and organizing data on the applicants and Fellows. The committee recommends that:

- USIP continue to collect the data for new applicants and fellows.
- USIP contact fellows to collect data currently missing from the spreadsheet.
- USIP collect new data to facilitate a better description of applicants and fellows. In particular, USIP could include a longer project description in the spreadsheet and could identify fellows as to whether they consider themselves to be scholars or practitioners.

Understanding How Fellows' Research Advances USIP and U.S. Foreign Policy Goals

For a number of reasons discussed in the report, the committee was not able to make much progress in meeting this part of its charge beyond presenting a basic overview of Fellows' research. To complete the second part of the committee's charge and to better interpret the findings above, the committee recommends the following strategy:

- USIP should conduct interviews or expert panels with former and current staff and board members to trace and assess the evolution of USIP's goals with respect both to the Fellowship program and the USIP mandate.
- USIP may wish to take a similar approach and collect information from external actors (e.g., government officials, academic experts, etc.). Although, ultimately, the program should be evaluated based on USIP's rationale, it would nevertheless be interesting to see how these actors judged the purpose of the fellowship. (A start at this approach is that both the survey of Fellows and the survey of peace and security experts included questions on this, as presented in Chapters 3 and 4.)
- USIP should take steps to identify U.S. foreign policy goals to see how the working of the program relates to broader U.S. foreign policy goals. The committee suggests that a strategy for accomplishing this would involve identifying important foreign policy challenges or goals and examining which of those areas Fellows are researching—both before and after these challenges or goals are identified by policymakers and other "thought leaders." This would enable USIP to begin to examine whether the research done under its aegis lags or leads larger policy issues.
- The survey findings also raise an issue about the purpose of the fellowship that could be further explored. Specifically, USIP should investigate whether to seek Fellows to advance thinking and offer more cutting-edge thinking in targeted areas, or focus on the application of such thinking to USIP priority issues.

Making Monitoring and Evaluation a Regular Part of the Fellowship

The committee feels strongly that USIP should undertake more rigorous and systematic monitoring and evaluation (M&E) of the Fellowship in the future. There are a number of approaches that USIP could take to develop a useful M&E strategy:

- Conduct an evaluation midway through the Fellowship to assess the match between resources and the Fellow's productivity, and to ascertain whether flexibility in timing and travel is needed.
- Hold an exit interview with all Fellows at the conclusion of the Fellowship. An interview could focus on such topics as:
    1. identify the various activities that Fellows pursued and how much time they spent on them.
    2. a list of Fellows' output, in particular asking what the Fellows believe to be their most important work. This could be done by collecting Fellow's CVs.
- Conduct an impact assessment of Fellows' work, completed during their Fellowship period. Ideally, such an approach would consist of (1) identifying all the products a Fellow produced during or directly related to the Fellowship, and (2) quantifying the impact of those works.

Conduct an impact assessment of the Fellowship on Fellows' careers. Once an initial assessment was undertaken, the process could be updated on a periodic basis. The committee suggests a number of possible directions that USIP might pursue.

Understanding External Perceptions of the Fellowship

The committee also makes several recommendations intended to help USIP gain further knowledge about the perceptions of the Fellowships in the wider expert community.

- USIP should continue to probe the external peace and security community about their perceptions of the program's impact. Information collected can assist USIP in reaching out to a broader audience, better tailoring its message, and improving competition for the fellowship by increasing the number of qualified applicants.
    1. Information collected should include topics from the survey of experts, as well as additional topics.
    2. Information should be collected from a broad range of experts, including academics, nongovernmental/nonprofit organization employees, and government employees.
- USIP should consider mixed modes to collect the data, reflecting the challenges of tapping different types of respondents' views.
- USIP's future research on the views of the expert community should seek more in-depth commentary on the impact of the program.

Improving the Fellowship Experience

Based on the survey results, the Committee recommends certain steps be considered to improve the Fellowship:

- Explore setting up an alumni network for former Fellows. Such a network could take advantage of the current USIP website or involve a new product,

for example by tapping a social network site. One way to facilitate a network would be to hold a meeting of Fellows designed to build such a network.
- Consider establishing support from businesses or associations in the community to help fellows and families cope with expenses of life in the D.C. area.
- Consider the potential for and ramifications of allowing for extensions of time to the Fellowship in individual cases. Some fellows and USIP may benefit greatly from having individual fellowships extended for a few months. In addition, USIP might want to consider greater flexibility in travel and support options for research outside DC, especially internationally, during the Fellowship.

Chapter 1
Overview

THE UNITED STATES INSTITUTE OF PEACE

The United States Institute of Peace (USIP) is an independent, nonpartisan, national institution established and funded by Congress. USIP was chartered under Sec. 1701 ("United States Institute of Peace Act") under Title XVII of the Defense Authorization Act of 1985.

The formal idea of a "peace office" dates back to 1792, when Benjamin Banneker and Dr. Benjamin Rush first proposed the establishment of a Peace Office.[1] In the twentieth century, a number of calls for the creation of a peace institute were made. From 1935 to 1976, more than 140 bills were introduced in Congress to establish various peace-related departments, agencies, bureaus, and committees of Congress.

In 1976, Sen. Vance Hartke of Indiana and Sen. Mark Hatfield of Oregon introduced a bill to create the George Washington Peace Academy. After hearings in the Senate on the Hartke-Hatfield Bill, it was decided that further study was needed. In 1979, a provision was successfully added to the Elementary and Secondary Education Appropriation Bill for the establishment of the Commission on Proposals for the National Academy of Peace and Conflict Resolution. A nonpartisan group consisting of appointees named by President Jimmy Carter and the leadership of the House and Senate, the Commission—chaired by Sen. Spark Matsunaga of Hawaii—worked for over a year and a half.

In 1981, after the completion of its deliberations, the Matsunaga Commission issued a final report recommending the creation of a national peace academy. Based upon the recommendations included in the report, bills were subsequently introduced in both houses of Congress under the bipartisan sponsorship of senators Mark Hatfield, Spark Matsunaga, and Jennings Randolph and Congressman Dan Glickman. Three years later, the United States Institute of Peace Act was finally passed and signed into law by President Ronald Reagan in 1984. USIP's Board of Directors was installed and held its first meeting in February 1986. In April of that same year, an initial staff of three people opened the Institute's first office.

The stated goals of the USIP are "to help:
- Prevent and resolve violent international conflicts
- Promote post-conflict stability and development
- Increase conflict management capacity, tools, and intellectual capital worldwide

The Institute does this by empowering others with knowledge, skills, and resources, as well as by directly engaging in peace building efforts around the globe."[2]

---

[1] The following material is taken from the USIP website. See also Montgomery (2003) and Weigel (1984/1985).
[2] From *About USIP* factsheet available at: http://www.usip.org/newsmedia/about_usip.pdf.

The USIP's overall focus has changed over the years. Perhaps the most substantive change had to do with the end of the Cold War (Wong 1993). In a speech in 2004 USIP Board Chairman Chester Crocker neatly summarized the evolution of issues during the USIP's existence.

Since its inception, the Institute has faced a changing context—just as the nature of international conflict constantly changes—and that context has helped the Institute broaden its reach and develop its capabilities. Think back to the events and issues that have been part of our working environment over the years:
- The end of the Cold War and the final collapse of empires.
- The rise of so-called ethnic conflict.
- The era of peacemaking in the Middle East…and its high-water mark in 1993.
- The ongoing debate on humanitarian intervention, and whether the United States should use force to advance its own values and those of the international community.
- How to professionalize peacekeeping and get it right, which was the precursor to today's debates about how to do post-conflict reconstruction and reconciliation, and about whether and how to do nation- or state-building.
- How to help stabilize and reconcile societies in transition—via programs in the fields of religion, rule of law, public security reform, educational reform, and through skills training in conflict management and problem-solving capabilities.

Crocker continued:

…September 11, 2001, and our ensuing engagement in coercive regime change is another watershed in the Institute's evolution. It produced the challenge of relating to post-conflict reconstruction and state building by offering our advisory services to local parties and to our own government at a time when the United States is at war—when we Americans are a direct party to the conflict and when we are in some sense a potential target (Crocker 2004).

Jennings Randolph Senior Fellows

The Jennings Randolph Program for International Peace was created at the same time as the USIP. The United States Institute of Peace Act notes that "The Institute, acting through the Board, may— (1) establish a Jennings Randolph Program for International Peace and appoint, for periods up to two years, scholars and leaders in peace from the United States and abroad to pursue scholarly inquiry and other appropriate forms of communication on international peace and conflict resolution and, as appropriate, provide stipends, grants, Fellowships, and other support to the leaders and scholars."

According to the USIP Web site:

The Jennings Randolph Program for International Peace awards Senior Fellowships to enable outstanding scholars, policymakers, journalists, and other professionals from around the world to conduct research at the U.S. Institute of Peace on important issues concerning international conflict and peace. The program integrates the work of Senior Fellows into the Institute's education, research, training, and operational activities. It also works closely with USIP's staff to disseminate knowledge from these projects to policymakers, researchers, educators, and the general public through a combination of policy briefings, public events, media appearances, and published materials—including books and reports. Since 1987, the Jennings Randolph Program has awarded over 200 Senior Fellowships and has established itself since its founding as one of the nation's premier Fellowship programs for research on international conflict management and peace building.[3]

Characteristics of the program include:
- Location: Fellows carry out their projects in residence at USIP in Washington, D.C.
- Duration: Fellowships are usually awarded for ten months, beginning in October. Shorter-term residencies are also available.
- Citizenship: Fellowships are open to citizens of any country. Many Jennings Randolph Senior Fellows are foreign nationals.
- Salary and benefits: The program attempts to match the income earned by the recipient during the year preceding the Fellowship, up to a maximum of $80,000 for ten months. The award covers health insurance premiums (80 percent), travel to and from Washington for Fellows and dependents, and a half-time research assistant. (The committee notes that although the cost of living in Washington, DC has risen in recent years, salaries for Fellows have not increased in some years.)

Applications are reviewed once per year; the submission deadline is in the Fall. Applicants to the Fellowship download the application form from the USIP Web site and submit their applications. For administrative purposes, USIP stores selected information from the applications in a database.

Fellows are selected through a rigorous, multi-stage review process that involves external reviewers, staff, and the USIP executive office and Board of Directors. Applications are first reviewed by staff. In particular, the USIP staff looks for areas of overlap between the research topic areas proposed by each applicant and USIP's current focus. The USIP staff comments on the applications at this stage. The applications are then sent out for external review by a panel of experts, including former Fellows. This process leads to a ranking of the applicants. Next, the applications are reviewed at the executive level of USIP. USIP board members conduct phone or face-to-face interviews with the applicants and pick primary and alternate candidates to receive the Fellowship. Finally, the full board votes on the slate. Offers are made to selected applicants; most accept, though in the past one or two have declined each year.

During their residency, Fellows are engaged with USIP in two ways: by generating products related specifically to their research or to their interests more generally, and by participating in USIP activities. As noted in the application:

> In keeping with its legislative mandate to support "scholarly inquiry and other appropriate forms of communication," the Jennings Randolph Program invites

---

[3] Available at http://www.usip.org/fellows/index.html.

proposals that would produce Institute publications. The editorial staff of the Institute works closely with Fellows to develop manuscripts for consideration by the Institute Press or for publication as Institute reports. Fellowship products may include the following:

- Books or monographs published by USIP Press;
- *Peaceworks* reports or Special Reports published by the Institute;
- Articles for professional or academic journals;
- Op-eds and articles for newspapers or magazines;
- Radio or TV media projects;
- Demonstrations or simulations;
- Teaching curricula;
- Lectures, workshops, seminars, symposia, or other public speaking.[4]

Additionally, Fellows may participate in various USIP activities. Some of these, such as giving lectures or briefings, overlap with these outputs. Of course, Fellows also take advantage of events that occur in Washington, such as attending Congressional hearings or lectures at other think tanks or nongovernmental organizations (NGOs), and networking with the many stakeholders in the area.

The program has received little attention in terms of an evidence-based evaluation of its merits and accomplishments.[5] USIP would benefit from a program evaluation in a number of ways. First, it would validate the benefits of the program by assessing the views of both participants and external observers. Second, it would facilitate greater efficiency in the process of disseminating information about the program, the application process, the selection process, and the experience of the Fellows. Third, it would facilitate greater effectiveness. Fourth, and finally, an evaluation would provide staff, other stakeholders, and potential Fellows with important information about the program.

THE COMMITTEE'S CHARGE

The National Research Council (NRC) appointed an ad hoc committee to conduct the assessment of the Jennings Randolph Program for International Peace Senior Fellowships (see Appendix A for committee member bios). The committee was asked to develop methodologies for conducting the assessment; to advise on data collection; to review data; to review findings about the Fellowship Program; and to provide recommendations for possible future assessments. The committee specifically addressed the following questions:
1. What are the characteristics of U.S. Institute of Peace (USIP) Senior Fellows and how have those characteristics changed over time?
2. What issues do Fellows research and how do those issues relate to the mandate of the USIP and to U.S. foreign policy?

---

[4] Available at http://www.usip.org/fellows/apply.html.
[5] An exception is Elise Boulding (1992). Boulding asks: "How well represented is the peace research and practitioner community among the fellows…?" She also examines the subject areas funded by USIP.

3. How do former Fellows and members of the external peace and security community perceive the program with respect to its:
    a. Impact on the Senior Fellows themselves;
    b. Advancement of the mandate of the USIP; and
    c. Contribution to increased knowledge or awareness of peace and security issues?

APPROACH AND SCOPE

There was overlap among the tasks outlined for the committe and information collected from one source (such as that provided by former Fellows) was applicable across multiple tasks. Sources of information included individuals and the work of former Fellows. In the case of individuals, three groups were relevant: former Fellows, experts in the peace and security community outside USIP, and USIP staff and board members. In discussions with USIP staff during the planning stages of this project it was decided that the committee would focus on just the first two groups.

As noted earlier, Fellows are involved in a number of outreach activities; these include producing written material (books, chapters, articles, special reports, and op-eds), giving briefings, lectures, or interviews, attending meetings, etc. For this reason, the committee focused largely on the written products produced by Fellows during their tenure at USIP. To help improve evaluations that USIP might wish to make in the future, in Chapter 5 the committee recommends some additional strategies for quantifying Fellows' activities in other realms.

For data collection, the committee turned to data collected by the USIP on its Fellows and on applicants to the Fellowship. In addition, the committee conducted a census of former Fellows—not all of whom could be reached, however, because USIP had lost touch with them over the years and neither the staff nor USIP was able to find new contact information. The committee also conducted a preliminary survey of experts in the peace and security community. Finally, the committee examined other data and literature related to the Fellowship. A summary of the approach of the study is found in Table 1-1.

Table 1-1 Summary of research questions, sources of information, and data collection techniques.

Research Question	Source	Data Collection Technique	Type of Data
What are characteristics of Senior Fellows?	Archival data provided by USIP	Data collected in applications and from Fellows	Quantitative
Fellows' research in larger context	Archival data provided by USIP	Data collected from Fellows	Quantitative
Perceived impact of the program on Fellows	Former Fellows	Survey	Quantitative and qualitative
Perceived impact of the program on USIP	Former Fellows; peace and security experts	Survey	Quantitative and qualitative
Perceived impact of the program on knowledge creation	Former Fellows	Survey	Quantitative and qualitative
Views about the program	Former Fellows; peace and security experts	Survey	Quantitative and qualitative

INFORMATION USED

As noted previously, the committee relied on several sources of information in conducting its evaluation. These included:
1. Data provided by USIP

USIP has some information on each Senior Fellow from the Program's inception in 1987 through 2007, as well as some information on applicants from 1997 through 2007.[6] The information is maintained in a spreadsheet format that facilitates display of the data and visual comparisons. The information that was collected for the Fellows is listed in Table 1-2:

---

[6] The names of applicants who did not receive a Fellowship were kept confidential from the committee.

Table 1-2 Data from USIP

Variable	Description
ID	A unique identifier assigned to each Fellow
Begin YR	Beginning year of Fellowship
FY	Fiscal year of Fellowship
Last Name	Last name of Fellow
First Name	First name of Fellow
Employer Type[a]	Type of employer
Sex	Gender of Fellow
Citizenship	Country of citizenship of Fellow
Citnew[b]	Citizenship (1 = U.S., 0 = other)
Highest Degree	Highest academic degree awarded
Project Title	Project title
Project Issue[c]	Topic of the project
Issue new[d]	Aggregated topic code
Project Region[e]	Region of the world that the project covered
Project Country	Names of countries the project covered

SOURCE: Spreadsheet provided by USIP

NOTES: [a] There are 11 employer codes: Academic/Research, Government, Diplomacy, NGO, Legal, Political Analysis/Consultancy, Journalism/Media, Business, Military, UN/IGOs, Other.

[b] The "Citnew" variable was created by staff based on the Citizenship variable.

[c] There are 29 codes for project issues: Conflict, Religious/Ethnic Conflict, Gender Issues, Terrorism/Political Violence, Cycles of Conflict, Conflict Management and Resolution (CMR), Conflict Prevention/Early Warning, Negotiation/Diplomacy, Peacekeeping, Post-Conflict Activities and Peacebuilding, Humanitarian Intervention, International Law/Rule of Law, Arms Control and Deterrence, Human Rights, International Organizations, United Nations, Refugees and Migration Issues, International Economics, Foreign Aid, Economic Development, Political Economies, Political Systems/International Relations, Democracy, Environment/Natural Resources, Communication, Media and Information Technology, Education, Foreign Policy, Other.

[d] The "Issue new" variable was created by staff by aggregating the codes for project issues into eight categories: conflict; conflict management/resolution; law, human rights, international organizations; economics and aid; political systems/democracy; environment, education/communication, foreign policy, and other.

[e] Ten geographic regions were identified: Western Europe, Eastern Europe/Former USSR, North America, Central and South America, Middle East/North Africa, Sub-Saharan Africa, East Asia, South Asia, Southeast Asia and Oceania, and Global.

*****

The committee used this information to examine characteristics among the Senior Fellows and applicants and compared selected characteristics of the two groups. Two issues are noteworthy: missing data and comparability. In general, there are very few missing data concerning basic statistics for the Fellows. One exception is the country or countries that the Fellow's research project addressed. There are no data for 147 out of 253 cases.

The gold standard for evaluating the impact of a program is a comparison of randomized groups. This would require USIP to identify those applicants who would be accepted to the program and randomly accept some of them and then compare these two groups. The purpose of the comparison is to identify measures of success (e.g., productivity) and compare those outcomes among the different groups. One point of making this comparison is to control for other factors that might explain particular outcomes. Unfortunately, this strategy was not possible at this time. Thus, the committee's approach to answering task 2 in the charge was to focus on *perceptions* of the impact of the program. The distinction is between being able to report that a Fellow was helped in her career by the program significantly more than someone who did not receive a Fellowship, as compared with former Fellows saying that the Fellowship helped their careers. The former is more rigorous and thorough, though the latter remains informative and interesting.

2. A survey of former Fellows

The committee conducted a survey of former Fellows. There were 246 former Fellows—seven of whom had been a Fellow twice—for a total of 253 Fellowships. Of the 246 former Fellows, 24 are known to be deceased. Efforts undertaken primarily by USIP, but supplemented by NRC staff, located working email addresses for 184 of the remaining 222 former Fellows (including 6 of the 7 Fellows who had been awarded two Fellowships). A survey questionnaire, which is reproduced in Appendix B, was sent to all former Fellows for whom there was a working email address. The survey was preceded by an invitation letter from USIP and followed up by two emails. The number of Fellowships awarded each year and the number of Fellows contacted are illustrated in Table 1-3.

Table 1-3 Number of Fellowships and number contacted by year of Fellowship.

Fellowship Year	Fellowships	Contacted
1987	8	3
1988	10	6
1989	11	7
1990	12	5
1991	9	4
1992	17	12
1993	12	7
1994	15	9
1995	15	12
1996	14	11
1997	16	13
1998	10	9
1999	15	9
2000	11	8
2001	13	12
2002	10	9
2003	13	13
2004	12	11
2005	11	11
2006	11	11
2007	8	8
Total	253	190

SOUCE: Spreadsheet provided by USIP; data tabulated by staff
NOTES: The 253 Fellows include seven who each had two Fellowships; the 190 Fellows contacted include 6 who each had two Fellowships.

3. A survey of peace and security experts

To answer the questions in the committee's charge, the committee sought to tap the opinions of experts in the areas of peace and security, conflict and conflict resolution. In so doing, the committee faced two challenges. First, defining a population of such experts is difficult. USIP's mission is quite broad, geographically and topically—as are the projects that Fellows work on. Thus, many individuals would seem to be relevant. A related issue is that since the purpose of contacting experts is to survey their opinions about the USIP Fellowship, it would be important to find individuals who knew something about USIP. A second challenge, once these individuals were identified, was to successfully interview them.

The committee considered three approaches: expert panels, telephone interviews, and a Web-based survey. Expert panels offer the advantage of allowing participants to explore topics in-depth during a face-to-face meeting. However, a distinct disadvantage for an initial foray into the perceptions of experts is that, given cost constraints, the panels would have had to meet in Washington, DC, and thus would have restricted the geographic range from which to draw experts. It can also be difficult to bring experts together to participate in a discussion. Telephone interviews resolved the issue about getting a wider range of experts' opinions, but these interviews were also seen as costly. In addition, there was some concern about reaching experts over the summer. The committee thus decided on a Web-based survey, which allowed it to contact many individuals quickly.

The committee put together a survey questionnaire (see Appendix C). To identify a population of experts from which a sample would be drawn, the committee turned to a list of academic centers and nonprofit organizations in the United States maintained by USIP.[7] This list was supplemented by searching the Web for additional centers. In addition, federal agencies, including the State Department, Department of Defense, U.S. Agency for International Development, and the U.S. Government Accountability Office, along with four Congressional committees (the Senate committees on Foreign Relations and Armed Services and the House committees on Foreign Affairs and Armed Services) were searched in order to find individuals with email addresses who could receive the survey.

The sample selected from this population was not random. At academic centers and NGOs, the focus was on individuals who were directors, deputy directors, or senior personnel. For government employees, the focus was not on directors but on desk officers and Congressional staff. Total sample size was 235. The survey was fielded in July and August 2008, with no follow-ups after the initial contact. The committee viewed the survey as a pilot to begin to conduct an assessment and the sample is acceptable for this reason. The survey results should not be extrapolated beyond the respondents, however. Further research would be needed to ascertain how widespread the respondents' perceptions are.

OUTLINE OF THE REPORT

The report is divided into three main chapters. Chapter 2 examines characteristics of Fellowship applicants and awardees. Ratios of awardees to applicants, as well as demographic characteristics, are examined. Particular attention is paid to the research interests of the Fellows. Chapter 3 focuses on the results of the survey of Fellows. The three areas examined are: (1) their activities and outputs during their Fellowship; (2) their views on the overall quality of the Fellowship, their satisfaction with the Fellowship, and whether their various expectations for the Fellowship were met; and (3) selected post-Fellowship characteristics, such as whether they have remained in contact with USIP. Chapter 4 focuses on the results of the survey of experts drawn from the peace and security community. This chapter examines these experts' familiarity with the Fellowship and the degree of prestige they associate with it. It also looks at experts'

---

[7] Available at http://www.usip.org/library/rcenters.html#us.

views on the importance of the work of the Fellows and of the Fellowship. Finally, Chapter 5 presents the committee's recommendations for overcoming the limitations in the data available for its assessment and for ensuring that monitoring and evaluation become a regular feature of the program in the future.

Chapter 2
Characteristics of Applicants, Fellows, and Research Topics

USIP began its Fellowship program in 1987. Each year, the Institute has selected between 8 and 17 Fellows (median of 12). As shown in Figure 2-1, a total of 253 Fellowships have been awarded from 1987 through 2007 (7 Fellows received two Fellowships).

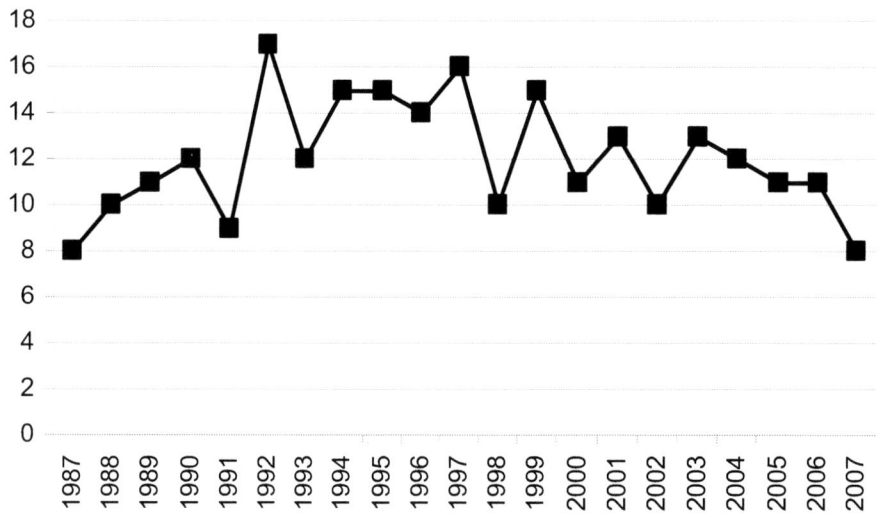

Figure 2-1 Number of Senior Fellowships awarded, 1987-2007
SOURCE: Data provided by USIP; tabulations by staff

An interesting question for USIP to consider is what the "right number" of Fellows is. This question draws attention to USIP's goals—to what degree is USIP seeking to support individuals as compared with creating a community of scholars and practitioners? Obviously, the answer is directly affected by USIP's resources.

USIP has only partial information on applicants to the program. For the period 1997-2007, USIP received 1,269 applications for Senior Fellowships. Yearly applications have ranged from 70 to 157, with a median of 120 (as shown in Figure 2-2).

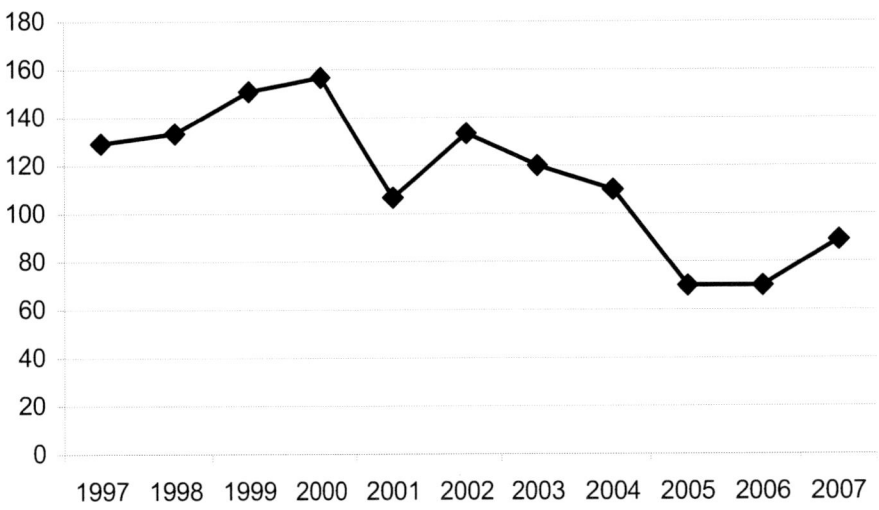

Figure 2-2 Number of applicants, 1997-2007
SOURCE: Data provided by USIP; tabulations by staff

Notice that the number of applicants appears to have dropped off when comparing the first five-year period to the latter five-year period. Future analysis could examine possible explanations for this trend. Possible explanations that could be tested include, among others: changes in the perception of the program; other opportunities for fellowships in peace and security; USIP efforts to reach out to potential applicants; changes in the overall labor market for potential fellows; and USIP's resources or goals.

From a competitiveness standpoint, USIP has many more applicants than positions (see Figure 2-3). The data collected by USIP, however, do not allow for analysis of the quality of individual applicants, so it is not clear from the information presented to the committee how many of these people would make good candidates for a Senior Fellowship.

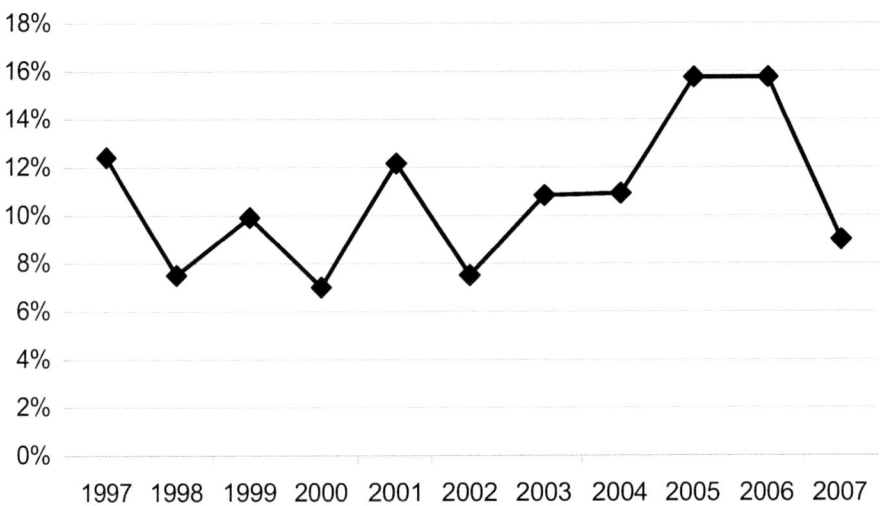

Figure 2-3 Ratio of number of Fellowships to applicants, 1997–2007
SOURCE: Data provided by USIP; tabulations by staff

Each year, USIP selects between 7 and 16 percent (mean of 11 percent) of applicants to become Fellows, and each year one or two of the individuals who are offered the Fellowship decline. Although the numbers are very small, it may be worthwhile for USIP to interview those individuals to ascertain why they declined the Fellowship. USIP could present them with specific choices, such as that the stipend was inadequate; they had pursued other, more attractive fellowships received simultaneously; or family or professional issues precluded their ability to relocate to Washington.

Additionally, further analysis could address such topics as:
1. What percentage of applicants is highly qualified for the Fellowship program?
2. What steps does USIP take to reach potential applicants? To what degree are their strategies effective?
3. Is the compensation adequate to attract a good pool of qualified applicants?
4. Should the competition be open to policy-relevant research across the board, or should the Fellows' research be tied more explicitly to USIP programming in the field?

An additional possibility would be to ask applicants how they heard about the program. Collecting information about this could assist USIP is improving its outreach to potential applicants.

DEMOGRAPHIC CHARACTERISTICS

Turning to demographic characteristics, USIP has collected data on the gender of Fellows and applicants and also on their citizenship. Regarding gender, 44 Fellows were women (17 percent where gender is known).[1] 302 applicants were women (24 percent

---

[1] There was 1 case where there was incomplete information on a Fellow, including that person's gender.

where gender is known).[2] Because the program selects few applicants per year, volatility in the percentage of particular groups of Fellows is to be expected. As can be seen in Figure 2-4, the percentage of female Fellows peaked in 1993, 2001, and 2006; it declined in 1998 and 2005.

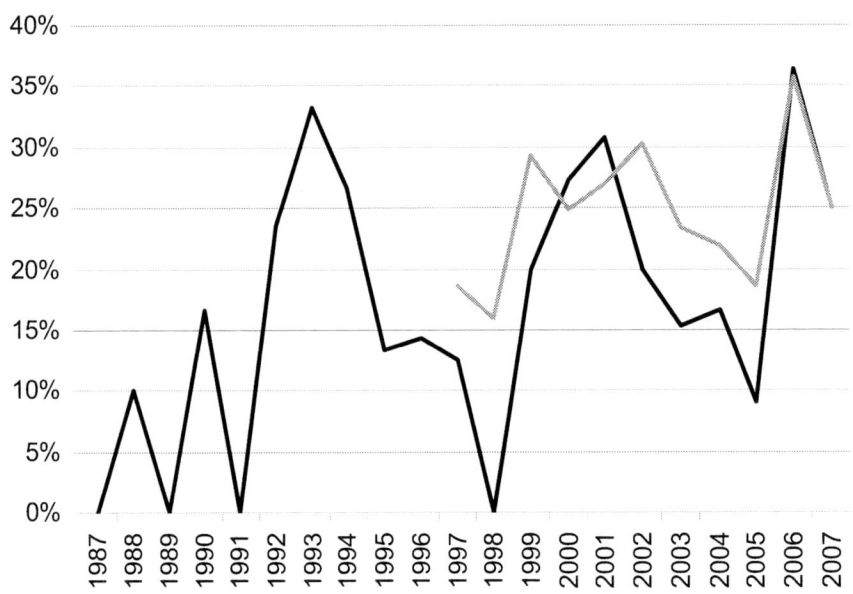

Figure 2-4 Percentage female Fellows, 1987-2007, and applicants, 1997-2007
SOURCE: Data provided by USIP; tabulations by staff

The percentage of women among the total number of applicants closely follows the percentage of women among the Fellows, except in 1998, and it assumes that the percentage of women accepting is similar to the percentage of men accepting Fellowship offers.

Forty-five percent of Fellows have U.S. citizenship (or dual-citizenship with the United States as one of the countries). The percentage of Fellows in any given year who are U.S. citizens varies widely, between 9 and 75 percent. Among applicants where citizenship is known, 30 percent have been U.S. citizens. As Figure 2-5 notes, a higher percentage of Fellows than applicants are U.S. citizens.

---

[2] There were 32 cases of missing data about gender.

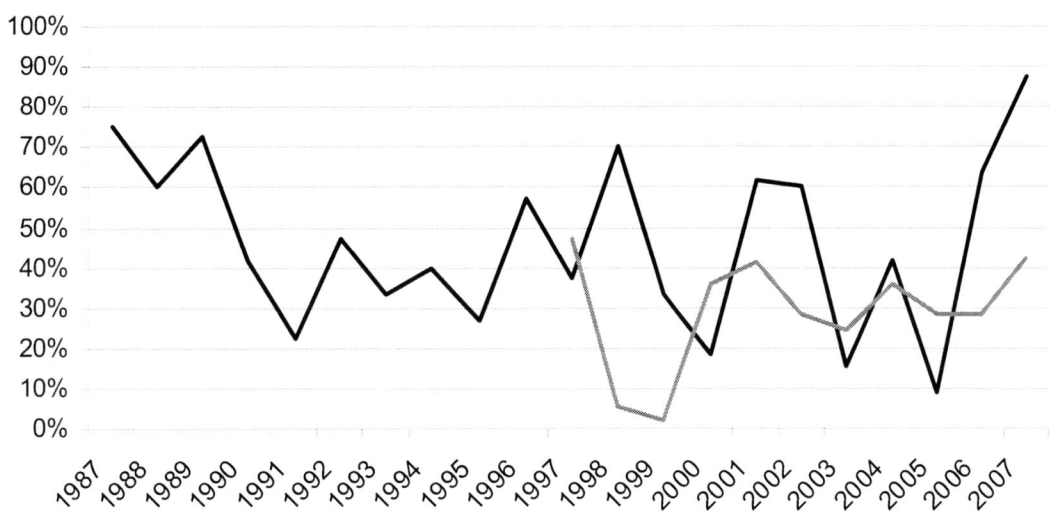

Figure 2-5 Percentage of Fellows, 1987-2007, and applicants, 1997-2007, who were U.S. citizens.
SOURCE: Data provided by USIP; tabulations by staff
NOTE: There are no missing data for the Fellows. There are missing data for the applicants. In particular, the drop in applicants who were U.S. citizens in 1998-1999 is due to missing data.

Among the countries from which the most non-U.S. applicants come are India, Nigeria, Israel, Russia, Pakistan, Canada, and the United Kingdom. Applicants have come from well over 100 different countries. Among the countries from which the most non-U.S. Fellows come are India, Israel, Russia, and the United Kingdom. Fellows have come from about 50 different countries.

Finally, we turn to a consideration of the employment of Fellows and applicants at the time of they applied for the Fellowship (as shown in Table 2-1).

Table 2-1 Type of employment of Fellows, 1987-2007, and applicants, 1997-2007

Type of Employment	Fellows	Percentage of Total	Applicants	Percentage of Total
Academic/Research	147	58	765	60
Government	29	11	97	8
Diplomacy	20	8	30	2
NGO	17	7	104	8
Legal	3	1	34	3
Political Analysis/Consultancy	5	2	40	3
Journalism/Media	19	8	82	6
Business	1	0	34	3
Military		0	12	1
UN/IGOs	6	2	17	1
Other		0	19	1
Missing	6	2	35	3
Total	253	100	1269	100

Source: Data provided by USIP; tabulations by staff

Overall, most of the applicants and Fellows are male, U.S. citizens, and academics. These demographic characteristics are noted for USIP, but no recommendation is made. It remains for USIP to determine what sort of demographic diversity fits with its goals for the Fellowship.

RESEARCH INTERESTS

The core of the Fellowship is a Fellow's research project. This section explores the thematic and geographic areas of the projects. As in the previous section, the foci are described. USIP can compare these trend data with its goals regarding which topics the institute would want to see Fellows address.

Subjects

USIP identified several foci of research projects that applicants propose, as noted in Table 2-2.

Table 2-2 Types of research foci

Major Category	USIP Categories
Conflict	Conflict
	Religious/Ethnic Conflict
	Gender Issues
	Terrorism/Political Violence
Conflict prevention, management, and resolution	Cycles of Conflict
	Conflict Management and Resolution (CMR)
	Conflict Prevention/Early Warning
	Negotiation/Diplomacy
	Peacekeeping
	Post-Conflict Activities and Peacebuilding
	Humanitarian Intervention
International law and organizations	International Law/Rule of Law
	Arms Control and Deterrence
	Human Rights
	International Organizations
	United Nations
	Refugees and Migration Issues
International economics	International Economics
	Foreign Aid
	Economic Development
	Political Economies
Political systems	Political Systems/International Relations
	Democracy
Environment and natural resources	Environment/Natural Resources
Communication	Communication
	Media and Information Technology
	Education
Foreign policy	Foreign Policy
Other	Other

As a starting point, these categories were collapsed into nine aggregated categories (as shown in Table 2-3): conflict; conflict prevention, management, and resolution; international law and organizations; international economics; political systems; environment and natural resources; communication; foreign policy; and other. It should be noted that, in the analysis that follows, the topics applicants pursued is partly influenced by the perceived focus of USIP; the topics that fellows pursued is partly influenced by the applicant pool and partly by the review committees that evaluated the applicants and recommended Fellows.

Table 2-3 Applicant research focus, 1997-2007

Year	Conflict	Conflict prevention, management, and resolution	Intl. law and orgs.	Intl. econ.	Political systems	Environ. and natural resources	Communication	Foreign policy	Other	Total
1997	17	45	23	7	20		12	4		128
1998	20	43	30	3	25	2	4	5	1	133
1999	25	45	26	10	27	1	8	8		150
2000	22	61	22	9	24	3	10	4	1	156
2001	17	37	16	3	26		5	3		107
2002	26	43	15	6	19	5	9	7	1	131
2003	24	33	22	1	25	2	6	4	2	119
2004	31	30	17	1	9	3	10	9		110
2005	18	27	11	2	6	1	2	2	1	70
2006	13	23	8	3	10	1	9	2	1	70
2007	27	23	13	2	15		8	1		89
Total	240	410	203	47	206	18	83	49	7	1263

SOURCE: Data provided by USIP; tabulations by staff

Looking at proportions of topics submitted annually by applicants, conflict represented between 13 and 17 percent from 1997 to 2001, then that topic rose from 2002 to 2007, peaking at about 30 percent in 2004 and 2007. Conflict prevention, management, and resolution topics averaged 34 percent of applicants' topics from 1997 to 2002 and 30 percent from 2003 to 2007. Minor trends—such as a drop-off in applications on topics related to political systems in 2004-2005 or the rise in topics related to communications in 2006-2007—also occurred, but largely the proportion of topics in each category has been fairly stable over time. Overall, conflict prevention, management, and resolution topics were the most common, followed by conflict, political systems, and international organization and law topics, as noted in Table 2-4.

Table 2-4 Applicant research focus by topic

Topic	Percentage
Conflict prevention, management, and resolution	32
Conflict	19
Political systems	16
International law and organizations	16
Communication	7
Foreign policy	4
International economics	4
Environment and natural resources	1
Other	1
Total applicants	1263

Source: Data provided by USIP; tabulations by staff

Similar analysis is presented for the research topics of Fellows in Table 2-5.

Table 2-5 Research topics of Fellows, 1987-2007

Year	Conflict	Conflict prevention, management, and resolution	Intl. law and orgs.	Intl. econ.	Political systems	Environ. and natural resources	Communication	Foreign policy	Other	Total
1987	2		2	1	2					7
1988	1	7	1				1			10
1989	1	6	1	1	2					11
1990	1	5	2	1				3		12
1991		3	4		1	1				9
1992	2	7	3	1	3			1		17
1993	4	4	1		3					12
1994	3	9			1		1	1		15
1995	3	3	1	1	5			2		15
1996	3	4	1	1	5					14
1997	3	6	2		3		2			16
1998	2	1	3		2	1	1			10
1999	3	5			5		1	1		15
2000	1	2	3	1	1	1	1			10
2001	2	5	4		1		1			13
2002		2	2	1	2	1		1	1	10
2003	2	3	2		3		1	1		12
2004	4	6	1				1			12
2005	4	4	2					1		11
2006	1	3	2		1		3	1		11
2007	2	1	2		2		1			8
Total	44	86	39	8	42	4	14	12	1	250

SOURCE: Data provided by USIP; tabulations by staff

Because of the limited number of Fellows annually, it is difficult to discern trends. One approach is to consider what the most frequent research topic was in a given year. In eight separate years—for instance in 1988 or again in 2004—the most frequent topic was conflict prevention, management, and resolution. In three years (1991, 1998, and 2000), international organizations and law was the most frequently researched topics among the Fellows. In 1996, political systems were popular. In the other years—for example in 2007—the topics were tied; one-quarter of the Fellows studied conflict, international organizations and law, and another quarter political systems. Overall, the same four research areas that were most popular among the applicants were most popular among the Fellows, as Table 2-6 illustrates.

Table 2-6 Research topics of Fellows by topic area

Topic	Percentage
Conflict prevention, management, and resolution	34
Conflict	18
Political systems	17
International law and organizations	16
Communication	6
Foreign policy	5
International economics	3
Environment and natural resources	2
Other	0
Total research topics	250

Source: Data provided by USIP; tabulations by staff

As the tables show, most applicants and Fellows focused primarily on one of four areas: conflict prevention, management, and resolution; conflict; political systems; and international law and organizations.

Geographic Focus

The geographic areas of focus that USIP identified are listed in Table 2-7.

Table 2-7 Geographic areas of focus

Geographic Region
Western Europe
Eastern Europe/Former USSR
North America
Central and South America
Middle East/North Africa
Sub-Saharan Africa
East Asia
South Asia
Southeast Asia and Oceania
Global

Tables 2-8 through 2-11 look at the geographic focus of applicants and Fellows. Table 2-8 examines applicants' proposed research and considers into which region(s) of the world their research topics best fit.

Table 2-8 Geographic focus of applicants' proposed research by year

Year	W. Europe	EE/FSU	N. America	C. and S. America	ME/N. Africa	Sub-Saharan Africa	E. Asia	S. Asia	SE Asia and Oceania	Global	Total
1997	12	19	7	4	12	13	10	7		45	129
1998	8	24	5	5	8	25	4	6	1	47	133
1999	5	29	3	3	19	20	11	18	3	37	148
2000	3	27	5	3	11	28	9	17	6	45	154
2001	1	22	1	2	5	17	5	9	3	41	106
2002	2	13	3	5	9	20	7	18	3	51	131
2003	3	8	5	2	12	24	5	11	1	47	118
2004	3	7	2	5	10	13	3	15	6	46	110
2005	4	9	2	2	15	7	2	11		17	69
2006	2	8		6	8	10	4	10	2	20	70
2007	2	7		7	25	8	4	9	2	25	89
Total	45	173	33	44	134	185	64	131	27	421	1257

Source: Data provided by USIP; tabulations by staff

The most frequent categorization in each year was "global," suggesting that applicants were approaching particular topics more generally (e.g., negotiation or diplomacy rather than diplomacy in the Middle East). Excluding this category, most applicants from 1997 to 2001 focused on Eastern Europe and the Former Soviet Union and sub-Saharan Africa. From 2003 to 2006, there was a relative shift in focus towards sub-Saharan Africa and South Asia. In 2007, topics about the Middle East and North Africa made up 28 percent of applicants' proposals. In general, these areas of the world were the most common in applicants' proposals, as Table 2-9 shows.

Table 2-9 Geographic focus of applicants' proposed research by percentage

Region	Percentage
Global	33
Sub-Saharan Africa	15
EE/FSU	14
ME/N. Africa	11
S. Asia	10
E. Asia	5
W. Europe	4
C. and S. America	4
N. America	3
SE Asia and Oceania	2
Total	1257

Source: Data provided by USIP; tabulations by staff

Similar tables were constructed for Fellows.

Table 2-10 Geographic focus of Fellows' research by year

Year	W. Europe	EE/FSU	N. America	C. and S. America	ME/N. Africa	Sub-Saharan Africa	E. Asia	S. Asia	SE Asia and Oceania	Global	Total
1987	1	2				1				3	7
1988	1			1	2	1				5	10
1989		2				2		2		5	11
1990		1		1	1		1	1		7	12
1991		1		1	3					4	9
1992		4			1	3		1		8	17
1993		1			1	4	1	1		4	12
1994		3		1	2	2	1	2		4	15
1995		4			3	1	1			6	15
1996	1	6		1		2	1			3	14
1997	1	3	1		4			2		5	16
1998		3			1	2	1			3	10
1999		5	1		4	1		1		3	15
2000		3	1		2		1			3	10
2001		1			2	1	1		1	7	13
2002		2				2	1	1		4	10
2003		2			3	1				6	12
2004		1			2	1		2	3	3	12
2005		2		1	3	1		2		1	10
2006		1		1	2	1	1	1		4	11
2007		1			5					2	8
Total	4	47	3	7	41	26	10	16	4	90	248

Source: Data provided by USIP; tabulations by staff

As the table shows, the work of many Fellows also fits within the "global" category. Focus on Eastern Europe and the Former Soviet Union seemed to peak from 1994 to 2000. Middle East and North Africa foci were popular from 1997 to 2001, and again from 2003 to 2007. (In particular most of the 2007 Fellows were working in this region). A general view echoing these trends is presented in Table 2-11.

Table 2-11 Geographic focus of Fellows' research by percentage

Region	Percentage
Global	36
EE/FSU	19
ME/N. Africa	17
Sub-Saharan Africa	10
S. Asia	6
E. Asia	4
C. and S. America	3
W. Europe	2
SE Asia and Oceania	2
N. America	1
Total	248

Source: Data provided by USIP; tabulations by staff

Excluding broadly international projects, applicants and Fellows generally focused on the same areas. This would seem to make sense in that if most applicants were proposing topics in the Middle East and North Africa, one would expect to see more Fellows doing research in that area. Looking at trends over time, applicants and Fellows alike have shown little interest in Southeast Asia and Oceania. Western Europe has been a declining focus among applicants and it has not been a focus for Fellows either. Eastern Europe and the Former Soviet Union also seemed to show a declining trend for both groups.

USIP did collect some data on specific countries of focus, but there are substantial missing data. For applicants, the countries that were most frequently proposed for study were China, India, Iraq, Israel/Palestine, Nigeria, Russia, South Korea, and the United States. Where Fellows focused on individual countries (in about half of the Fellows' projects), the most frequently studied places were Russia, China, Iran, Iraq, and Israel/Palestine. It is likely that some of the country focus is explained by conflicts that are occurring in or involving those particular countries. As conflict shifted over time from the 1980s to the 2000s, it is likely that the interests of applicants and USIP would change and that this would be somewhat reflected in the work of the Fellows.

FINDINGS

In response to the first question in the committee's charge, and based on the data provided by USIP, the committee found:
1. USIP's data spreadsheet is a useful organizing tool.
2. Each year, USIP selects between 7 and 16 percent (mean of 11 percent) of applicants to become Fellows (Figure 2-3), which could indicate the program is very competitive.

3. Most Fellows and applicants are male and academics. Seventeen percent of Fellows are female (where gender is known).On average 45 percent were U.S. citizens (Figures 2-4, 2-5, Table 2-1).
4. Overall, conflict prevention, management, and resolution were the most common topics for Fellows and applicants, followed by conflict, political systems, and international organization and law topics, (Tables 2-3, 2-4, 2-5, and 2-6).
5. In terms of geographic focus, many Fellows work fit into the "global" category. Focus on Eastern Europe and the Former Soviet Union seemed to peak from 1994 to 2000. The Middle East and North Africa foci were popular from 1997 to 2001, and from 2003 to 2007 (in particular most of the 2007 Fellows were working in this region). Research on sub-Saharan Africa ranked fourth among the areas of geographic focus for Fellows' research (Tables 2-10, 2-11).
6. Applicants took a somewhat different approach; after global projects, sub-Saharan Africa was the subject of the most proposals, followed by Eastern Europe and Soviet Union/Former Soviet Union, the Middle East/North Africa, and South Asia (Tables 2-8, 2-9).

Chapter 3
Views of Former Fellows

One of the key steps in the assessment of the Jennings Randolph Senior Fellowship was to survey former Fellows. The survey was sent to 184 out of 246 former Fellows.[1] One hundred sixteen Fellows responded to the survey, a response rate of about 63 percent (the distribution of survey responses is shown in Table 3-1).

Table 3-1 Distribution of respondents by year of Fellowship

Fellowship Year	Fellows	Contacted	Responded
1987	8	3	1
1988	10	6	3
1989	11	7	4
1990	12	5	4
1991	9	4	2
1992	17	12	4
1993	12	7	3
1994	15	9	4
1995	15	12	8
1996	14	11	10
1997	16	13	9
1998	10	9	4
1999	15	9	6
2000	11	8	4
2001	13	12	6
2002	10	9	10
2003	13	13	5
2004	12	11	7
2005	11	11	7
2006	11	11	4
2007	8	8	8
Total	253	190	113

SOURCE: Survey of former Fellows; data tabulations by staff.
NOTES: The number contacted includes six fellows who had each received two fellowships. The total number under the "responded" column excludes three Fellows who did not answer this question. One Fellow appears to have entered the wrong year in 2002.

Two possible sources of error in surveys are unit non-response (that is, some individuals who were sent the questionnaire do not respond, and their responses would

---

[1] The remaining Fellows could not be reached; some were deceased and some could not be located.

have differed significantly from the responses of those who did respond) and item nonresponse (respondents do not answer all the questions). The former is a concern in the committee's efforts to conduct a census of former Fellows. USIP did not have contact information for all Fellows. It is likely that Fellows who have "dropped off the radar" also have had less interaction with USIP. It may be that they also have different views about the Fellowship Program. Likewise, as noted previously, a number of Fellows who were contacted did not respond. These Fellows might also have different views. This potential nonresponse error should be considered in the following discussion of findings from the respondents. In all cases, findings are relevant only to the respondents and should not be extrapolated to USIP Fellows as a whole. Concerning item nonresponse, most respondents answered almost all questions; therefore, it does not appear that this is a source of error in the findings presented below. Throughout the survey, item nonresponse was between 1 and 9 percent; in other words, between 105 and 115 respondents answered individual questions. For many questions, only one respondent failed to answer the question.

ACCOMPLISHMENTS DURING THE FELLOWSHIP

First, the committee asked what sort of professional activities Fellows had engaged in during their Fellowship. The question was worded: "During your Fellowship, did you engage in any of the following professional or career development activities (check all that apply)?" As Figure 3-1 illustrates, the most frequent response was attending workshops, lectures, or seminars in the Fellow's research area. As the data show, Fellows were very engaged during their residency, with many of them selecting all four activities.

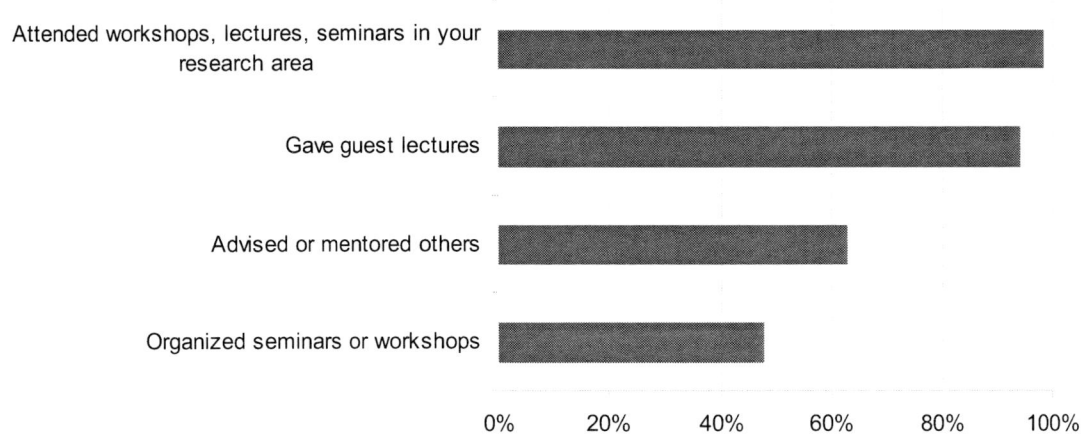

Figure 3-1 Percentage of respondents reporting professional or career development activities.
SOURCE: Survey of former Fellows; data tabulations by staff.
NOTE: n = 115.

In addition, as shown in Table 3-2 respondents were given the opportunity to mention other activities. Seventeen respondents identified other activities, although many of those would fall into the category of workshops and meetings. A few, however, mentioned giving media interviews, one mentioned advocacy on Capitol Hill, and one mentioned training diplomats.

We then compared recent former Fellows to the earlier period of the program to see if there were any differences. One hundred thirteen respondents gave the year of their Fellowship. They were aggregated into two groups: 1987 to 2001 and 2002 to 2007. It was hypothesized that there might be some difference in the Fellows' experiences or views prior to and after the September 11th, 2001 terrorist attacks. This might be the result of a changed climate in Washington, DC; international scholars studying in the United States; focus on terrorism; a continued shift to a focus on non-state actors, etc.

Table 3-2 Percentage of respondents reporting professional or career development activities by year of Fellowship.

Activity	1987-2001	2002-2007
Gave guest lectures	93%	95%
Advised or mentored others	61%	63%
Organized seminars or workshops	50%	46%
Attended workshops, lectures, seminars in your research area	97%	98%
Number of Fellows	72	41

SOURCE: Survey of former Fellows; data tabulations by staff.

Fellows in both groups were quite similiarly involved in activities.

Second, the committee asked about the activities in which the Fellows engaged. The question was worded: "During your Fellowship, which of the following activities did you engage in (check all that apply)?" More than half of respondents gave guest lectures, gave media interviews, conducted research aside from their proposed research project, appeared on TV or radio talk shows, and wrote book manuscripts.

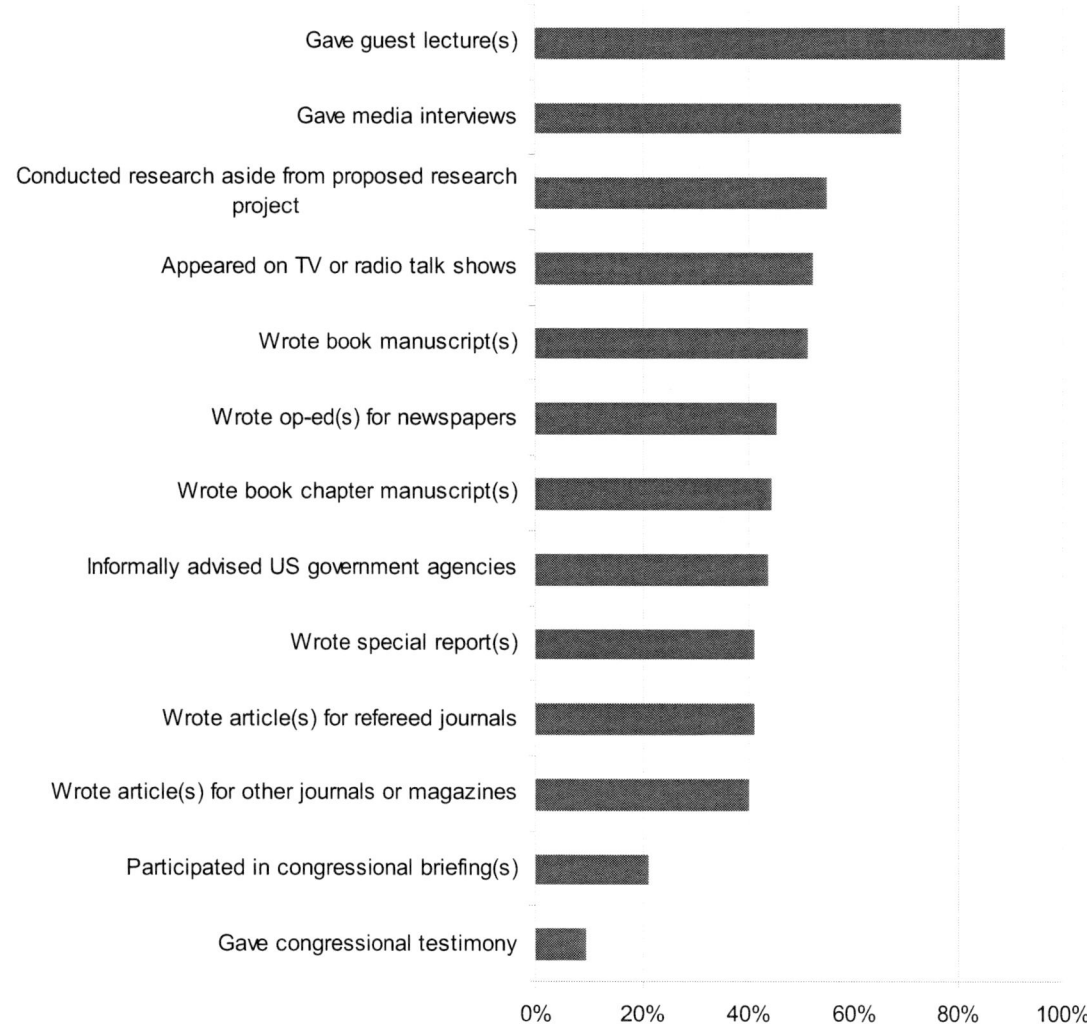

Figure 3-2 Percentage of respondents reporting engagement in activities, by type.
SOURCE: Survey of former Fellows; data tabulations by staff.
NOTE: n = 115.

One interesting finding was that a majority of Fellows also conducted research outside of their main area of research during their residency at USIP.

The committee then considered whether Fellows in more recent years engaged in different types of productive output than their counterparts in earlier years. Table 3-3 looks at various research and written products comparing the Fellows from the two time periods.

Table 3-3 Percentage of Fellows engaging in various measures of productivity by year of Fellowship.

Activity	1987-2001	2002-2007
Conducted research aside from proposed research project	54%	59%
Wrote article(s) for refereed journals	43%	39%
Wrote article(s) for other journals or magazines	39%	41%
Wrote special report(s)	39%	44%
Wrote book manuscript(s)	49%	56%
Wrote book chapter manuscript(s)	44%	44%
Number of Fellows	72	41

SOURCE: Survey of former Fellows; data tabulations by staff.

As Table 3-3 shows, Fellows in more recent years may be producing more products, as a higher precentage of these Fellows were conducting additional research, writing articles for non-referreed journals, writing special reports, and preparing book manuscripts. However, the survey does not allow for a definitive answer, since it measures neither quantity within a category (number of articles produced by a Fellow) nor quality. Additionally, there are direct and indirect impacts of the Fellows' work. Future research would be needed to address these impacts. Moreover, the survey does not shed light on whether this potentially greater output of Fellows is positive or negative for the Fellow or USIP. A future direction for assessment could be to undertake an analysis of resumes/curricula vitae to identify what Fellows produce (e.g., articles, books, presentations, etc.) during their Fellowship and related to the Fellowship, as compared with other output before and after their stay at USIP.

Table 3-4 focuses specifically on the outreach activities of the more recent Fellows compared with the earlier Fellows. As Table 3-4 shows, more recent Fellows have participated more in media outreach, but less than earlier Fellows in interacting with Congress. (An important note on both of these activities is that they are likely to be initiated by the media and Congressional staff and those requests probably go through USIP staff to Fellows. It is possible that changes in staff handling such requests has influenced how often Fellows engage in these activities.)

Table 3-4 Percentage of Fellows engaging in various activities by year of Fellowship

Activity	1987-2001	2002-2007
Wrote op-ed(s) for newspapers	43%	49%
Gave guest lecture(s)	89%	88%
Gave media interviews	64%	76%
Appeared on TV or radio talk shows	47%	59%
Participated in Congressional briefing(s)	22%	17%
Gave Congressional testimony	11%	7%
Informally advised U.S. government agencies	43%	44%
Number of Fellows	72	41

SOURCE: Survey of former Fellows; data tabulations by staff.

It may be instructive in future assessments to consider whether Fellows' opportunities to interact with Congress are declining and what this might mean for USIP's ability to bring important research to the attention of Congress, or whether Fellows in recent years are less interested in interacting with Congress.

VIEWS ABOUT THE FELLOWSHIP

Overwhelmingly, the respondents had a high regard for the program, as noted in Figure 3-3. Two-thirds of respondents selected "excellent."

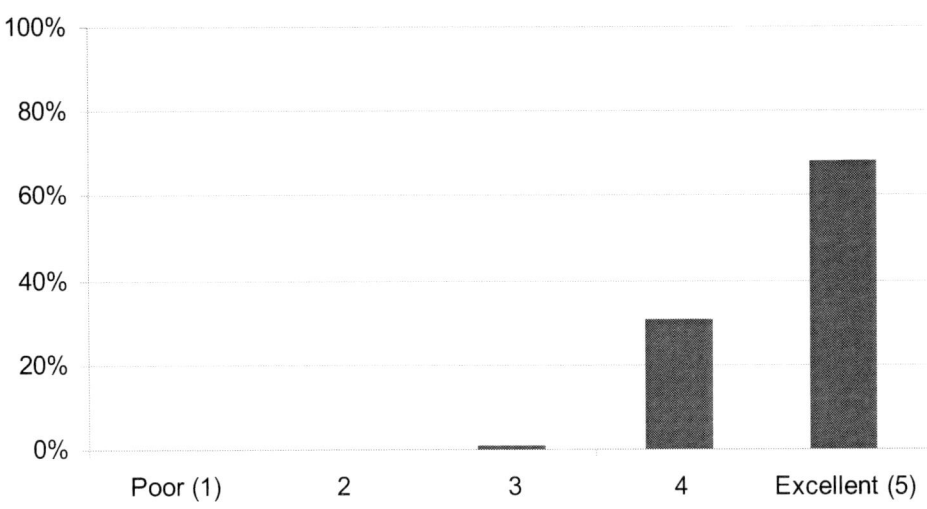

Figure 3-3 Respondents' perception of the overall quality of the Fellowship program
SOURCE: Survey of former Fellows; data tabulations by staff.
NOTE: n = 114.

The same is true for Fellows in earlier years versus those in more recent years, shown in Table 3-5.

Table 3-5 Respondents' perception of the overall quality of the Fellowship program by period of Fellowship

Fellow	Poor (1)	2	3	4	Excellent (5)	Total
1987-2001	0%	0%	1%	27%	71%	70
2002-2007	0%	0%	0%	39%	61%	41

SOURCE: Survey of former Fellows; data tabulations by staff.

Although earlier Fellows were more likely than later Fellows to assess the program as excellent, the percentage difference in Table 3-5 is not statistically significant at the 0.05 level.

The survey next asked what was the most important product that the Fellows had produced during their Fellowship. Overwhelmingly, the response was a written product, most frequently a book or book manuscript, book chapter(s), article(s), or special reports. Very few responses deviated from this trend, though a few did and are noteworthy. Two respondents noted that they had been able to convince policymakers to take action regarding conflicts that were occuring in Europe. Two respondents mentioned op-eds or media products. One respondent mentioned a blog (and commented that "it doesn't fit within the USIP framework of products"). One respondent complimented the research assistance at USIP in helping him prepare a lecture series. Several resondents mentioned specific research projects that were started at USIP during the Fellowship. A follow-up question in further research to start to get at quality and content issues could be to ask the Fellows, in their view, what was it about their work that made it so important.

The next question focused on whether the Fellowship met the expectations of the Fellow across a number of dimensions. As Figure 3-4 shows, there was a high degree of concurrence between what USIP provided and what Fellows expected, in particular, in such areas as the Fellows' ability to conduct their own research, access to research facilities and resources, ability to attend conferences, meetings, etc., and administrative support from USIP. Areas where there might be room for improvement lie in mentoring or advising and the Fellows' ability to collaborate with others at USIP.

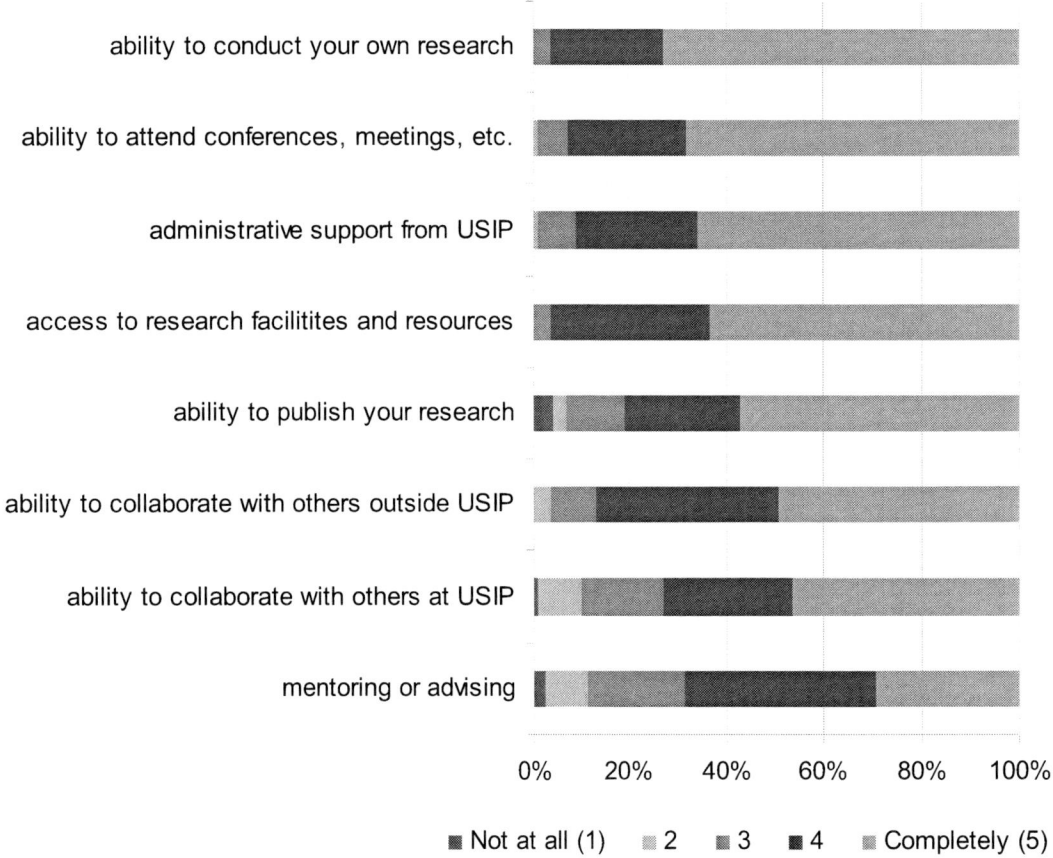

Figure 3-4 Degree to which Fellowship met Fellows' expectations by program aspect.
SOURCE: Survey of former Fellows; data tabulations by staff.
NOTE: 115 respondents answered at least part of this question, but some respondents left some choices blank, so for an individual choice (e.g., "ability to publish your research") the sample size ranged between 106 and 115.

Since mentoring was the area where Fellows' expectations were least met, the committee explored whether this might have been more of an issue more with earlier Fellows than with more recent ones. The results as noted in Table 3-6 are unclear.

Table 3-6 Degree, by year of Fellowship, to which Fellows' expectations regarding mentoring or advising were met

Fellow	Not at all (1)	2	3	4	Completely (5)	Hard to judge	Total
1987-2001	0%	8%	20%	30%	26%	17%	66
2002-2007	5%	8%	13%	37%	21%	16%	38

Source. Survey of former Fellows; data tabulations by staff.

Since the Jennings Randolph Fellowships are *senior* fellowships, it is not clear how much mentoring USIP should provide or what the nature of such mentoring should be. It is also not clear from the survey whether Fellows expected a lot or a little mentoring in absolute terms.

Next, the survey asked how useful the Fellowship was in enhancing the career of Fellows. As to be expected, the largest benefit was in increasing the Fellows' knowledge in the area of their Fellowship research project (see Figure 3-5). Almost 100 percent found the Fellowship quite useful (a score of 4 or 5 on a scale of 1 to 5) in this regard. Very positive results were also noted in terms of increasing a Fellow's network of colleagues. Among the four areas, the least useful one was the role of the Fellowship in improving a Fellow's research skills. (Of course, senior Fellows presumably already have good research skills.)

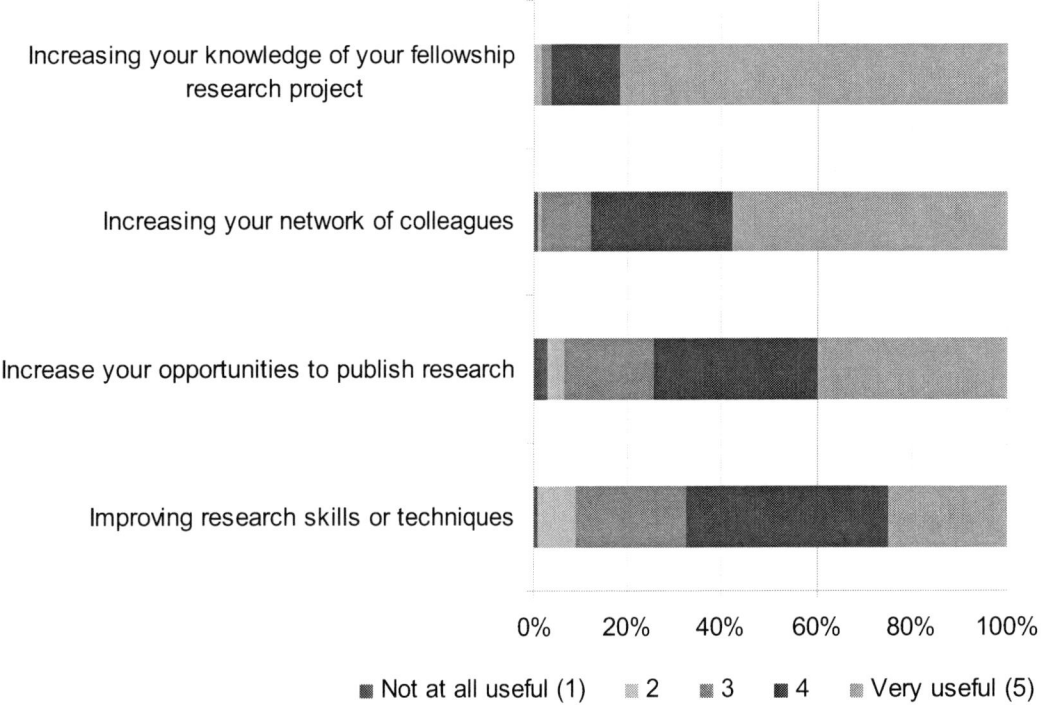

Figure 3-5 Degree of usefulness of Fellowship for Fellow, by aspect.
SOURCE: Survey of former Fellows; data tabulations by staff.
NOTE: n = 115.

We then looked specifically at networking (see Table 3-7). While a handful of recent Fellows did not find the Fellowship helpful in increasing their network of colleagues, most found the Fellowship very useful. Although the survey could not provide further insight into this result, it is possible that local Fellows and policy Fellows, as opposed to those farther from Washington, DC and academics, may have had less need of using USIP to develop their networks.

Table 3-7 Percentage of respondents, by period of Fellowship, who agreed that the Fellowship was useful in increasing network of colleagues

Fellow	Not at all useful (1)	2	3	4	Very useful (5)	Total
1987-2001	0%	1%	11%	34%	53%	70
2002-2007	3%	0%	8%	23%	68%	40

SOURCE: Survey of former Fellows; data tabulations by staff.

Focusing on a Fellow's network, the next question asked: "To what extent did your Fellowship provide you with the opportunity to interact with the peace and security community?" Considering scores of 4 and 5 (a great deal), Fellows were most likely to network with academics and practitioners. As can be seen in Figure 3-6, the least amount of interaction was with the media.

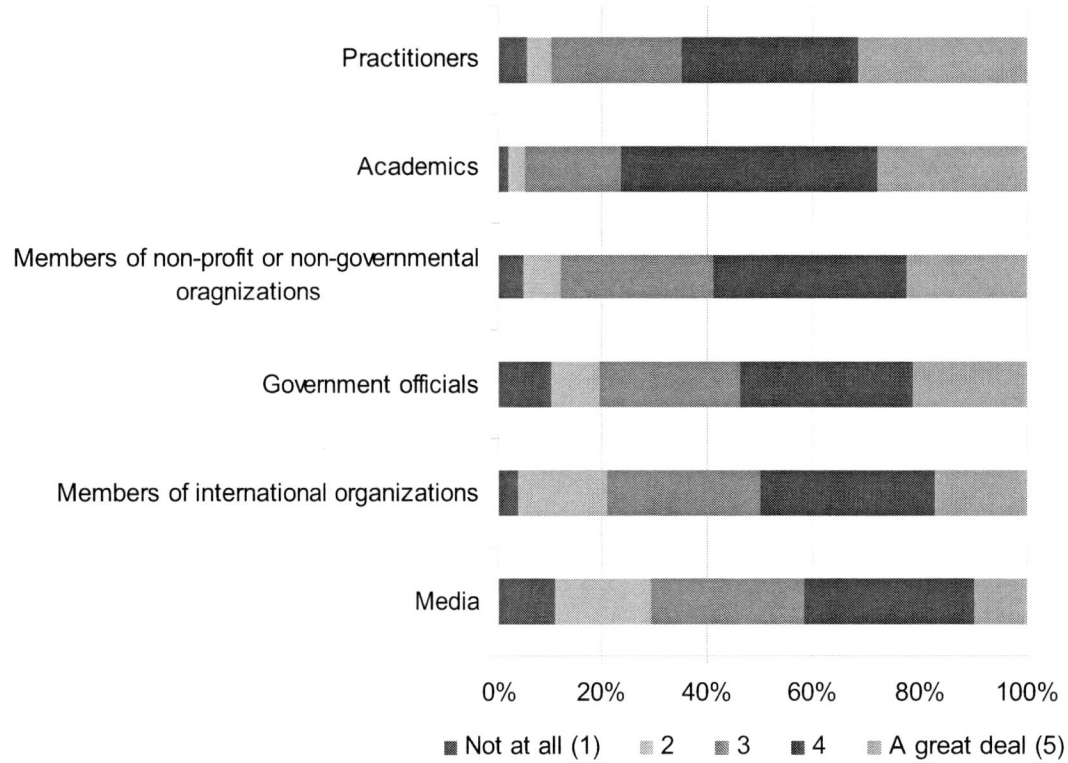

Figure 3-6 Extent of opportunity to interact with various networks.
SOURCE: Survey of former Fellows; data tabulations by staff
NOTE: n = 115.

The finding that Fellows seemed to have fewer interactions with the media at first seems at odds with the findings in Figure 3-2 that about 52 percent of Fellows appeared on TV or radio talk shows and 69 percent gave media interviews. Presumably, Fellows mean a different kind of interaction vis-à-vis this question. Here, too, it would be instructive to correlate the results in Figure 3-6 with the position of the individual Fellow (e.g., did academic Fellows interact with practitioners) and perhaps this can be done in future research.

Congress set the Fellowship's duration at up to two years, but in practice it has been ten months. Given the large amount of work Fellows do during their tenure, one might think that they would feel this period is too short. On the other hand, however, Fellows are taking sabbaticals from other positions (such as being a professor) and may want to get back to their full-time jobs. The survey asked respondents whether they considered ten months to be an appropriate amount of time for the Fellowship. A majority of respondents said it was, as noted in Figure 3-7.

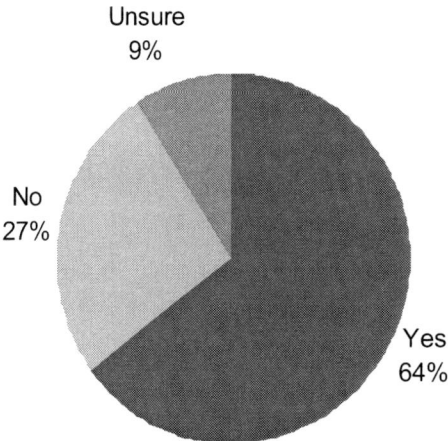

Figure 3-7 Percentage of respondents who agreed that ten months is the right duration for the Fellowship
SOURCE: Survey of former Fellows; data tabulations by staff.
NOTE: n = 113.

It should be noted that many Fellows are academics and a ten-month duration fits well with an academic calendar. This might explain why so many Fellows responded that ten months was about right. In the future USIP might ask during an exit interview with Fellows whether they thought they had had enough time to conduct their research. USIP might then disaggregate these data by the employment status of the Fellow. Among earlier Fellows who responded to that same question, 70 percent said yes, 23 percent said no, and the remaining respondents (7 percent) were unsure (n = 71). Among Fellows in more recent years, only 56 percent said yes, 33 percent said no, and the remaining respondents (10 percent) were unsure (n = 39).[2] The survey asked those who said no to elaborate. The most frequent response among those who thought more time was needed was 12 months, though a few said less time was needed (e.g., six months), and a few said

---

[2] Does not equal 100 percent because of rounding.

even longer was needed (up to two years). In thinking about its recruitment of future Fellows, USIP may want to seek more information about why fewer recent Fellows (although still a clear majority) think that ten months is the right length of time. A related point would be to ask former Fellows if they completed their project in the time allotted. One could also ask former Fellows how soon after they completed their Fellowship did they submitted their work for publication.

At this point, the survey asked respondents to describe the best and worst features of the program. Respondents consistently focused on a few basic themes, which are summarized in Table 3-8.[3] It should be underscored that only half of the respondents chose to fill this question out, and several who did wrote some variation of "nothing." In addition to the comments in Table 3-8, some respondents commented on the library, which they felt had inadequate access to information—though the reference point seems to be that of a university library, which often has very good access. Some respondents felt that they would have liked to receive more help in editing/publishing the results of their projects.

---

[3] Comments were edited for spelling and identifying information was removed. In a few cases, "[ ]" were added to provide clarifying terms.

Table 3-8 Major themes and examples of respondents' views of best and worst features of the Fellowship

Best feature of the Fellowship	"The best feature of the Fellowship was the chance it afforded to focus on research and writing, free from day-to-day academic duties." "To be able to write a book, and for the entire family to be able to become part of American society for almost a whole year." "Ability to concentrate on the project; interacting, exchanging ideas and information with other Fellows; supportive environment within the USIP." "The chance to meet with and learn from a talented and diverse group of professionals—both Fellows and Institute staff."
Worst feature of the Fellowship	**Perception of unequal demands on Fellows' time** "The pull to participate in other events related to your research, that distracted from research/writing." "The unequal demands made on Fellows: some, like myself, were asked to actively participate and work with USIP Programs, at times to the detriment of their own work…; others were free to do as they pleased and appeared to have few, if any, demands made on them by the Institute; indeed, they were hardly ever in their offices, which also meant very little opportunity for colleague-to-colleague discussions." **Amount of stipend, lack of resources for travel, and other financial issues** "Living in an expensive town on a tight budget." "The lack of a supplementary budget for things like conference attendance, field visits, and presentations." **Lack of engagement** "Isolation from other Fellows and some staff." "Lack of community, people to learn from at USIP in my subject area." "Limited occasions for just the Fellows and program staff to interact as a group."

Finally, the survey asked respondents "In what ways do you think the work you did during your Fellowship was helpful to USIP?" To reiterate from Chapter 1, the goals of USIP are "to help

- Prevent and resolve violent international conflicts.
- Promote post-conflict stability and development.
- Increase conflict management capacity, tools, and intellectual capital worldwide.

The Institute does this by empowering others with knowledge, skills, and resources, as well as by directly engaging in peacebuilding efforts around the globe."[4] Respondents

---

[4] From *About USIP* factsheet available at: http://www.usip.org/newsmedia/about_usip.pdf.

offered a few ways that they thought their time at USIP might assist USIP in meeting this mandate. A number of respondents focused on how they were spreading knowledge and informing various audiences.

> "Helped USIP to achieve visibility in my research areas…Opened up new contacts for USIP with the UN."

> "It provided up to date data and in-depth analysis of one of the most troubling conflicts currently high on the U.S. and international agenda. Promoted USIP's vision among policymakers and the academic community."

> "My work was focused on [name of topic] at the most critical time: I testified before Congress, briefed numerous members of Congress, appeared on CNN, Newshour, and numerous other [media] stations."

> "I provided media attention to USIP activities through interviews in CNN, CNBC, PBS and many other newspapers and radios. I also researched on a conflict that USIP had never covered before."

> "I presented papers at major conferences as a representative of the USIP. I increased its visibility."

Some Fellows felt that their work added to USIP's credibility.

> "My work provided knowledge of my research findings to USIP Fellows, to others coming to USIP meetings, and to the public. By receiving rave reviews, my book also added to the USIP's credibility as a funder of important, well-done research projects."

> "May have helped establish USIP credibility for supporting work on resolution of internal conflicts."

> "My research, including the survey data that I compiled while a USIP Fellow, has had an important impact in the 15 years since my Fellowship; along with subsequent projects USIP has funded, I believe it helped to put USIP on the map of important players in both the region and issues addressed in my research, many of which had not been addressed in USIP grants previously."

Fellows also thought that their time at USIP added depth to USIP.

> "My Fellowship was helpful to USIP to learn more about little known Central Asia."

> **"My research and book provided the USIP with an insight into the South African peace process which it would otherwise not have had."**
>
> **"I think I brought a South Asia perspective to the USIP's work."**
>
> **"It helped round out USIP's profile in an area that it hasn't specialized in."**
>
> **"Enabled Institute to get established in a region not well covered otherwise."**

Finally, several Fellows thought their work had a more direct effect on conflict resolution.

> **"I established linkages for the [name of group] with groups in the [name of country] who were all involved in securing peace and transforming conflict: government agencies – including…government officials, academe, civil society. I even invited Senator [name of individual] to speak at the Institute. I believe I was able to provide the USIP with inputs that led to their involvement as facilitator in the [name of country] government's peace process with the [name of group]. Before Ambassador [name of individual] became US Ambassador to the [name of country], I already had discussions with him about [name of subjects]. I continued the networking with Amb. [name of individual] when he assumed his post. He later recommended that USIP be tapped to help in the peace process."**
>
> **"This will give away my identity but I think I helped USIP make a contribution to bridging [names of parties] differences in the midst of their then ongoing border war."**

The next set of questions focused on the lasting impact of the Fellowship on the Fellows. First, the survey asked: "Do you continue to conduct research or work in the areas that your research project focused on?" Almost all respondents—112 out of 115 (97 percent)—indicated that they did. The remaining 3 percent reported not applicable (presumably, they were retired). This is an area where nonresponse bias might be particularly noteworthy, since Fellows who could not be reached might be less likely to be conducting research or to be working in the areas on which their research project focused. Thus, this percentage might be higher than what one might expect if one could have surveyed all Fellows.

The survey then asked to what extent former Fellows maintained relations with other Fellows or USIP staff and continued to participate in USIP activities. As Figure 3-8 shows, a majority of former Fellows have continued to stay in touch with both other Fellows and with USIP staff and to participate in USIP events.

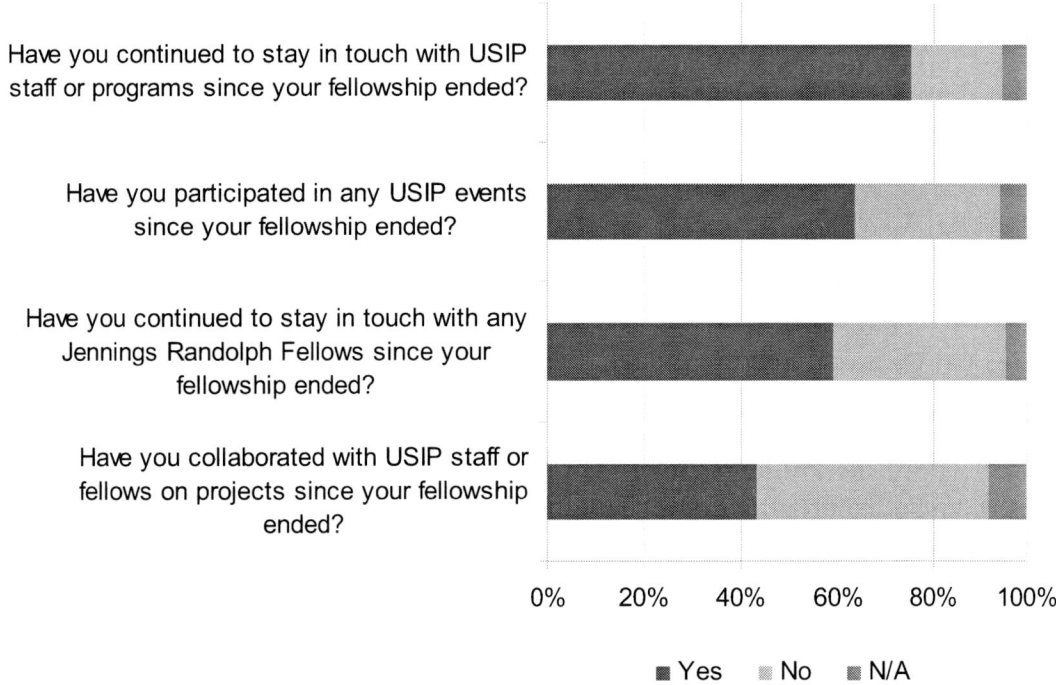

Figure 3-8 Post-Fellowship activities
SOURCE: Survey of former Fellows; data tabulations by staff.
NOTE: Sample sizes differ slightly. They are from top to bottom: 113, 112, 110, and 112.

There is a bit of a potential bias upward here, however, in that former Fellows for whom USIP had contact information were also probably more likely to stay in touch with USIP staff or to attend USIP events. This is also an area where there might be some differences based on when Fellows held their Fellowships. Focusing on those who said "yes" as a percentage of those who said "yes" or "no,"—that is, excluding Fellows who replied "not applicable"—Table 3-9 compares Fellows' post-fellowship activities by period of Fellowship.

Table 3-9 Fellows' post-Fellowship activities by year of Fellowship

Post-Fellowship activities	1987-2001	N	2002-2007	N
Have you continued to stay in touch with USIP staff or programs since your Fellowship ended?	78%	69	80%	35
Have you continued to stay in touch with any Jennings Randolph Fellows since your Fellowship ended?	61%	69	63%	35
Have you participated in any USIP events since your Fellowship ended?	74%	68	55%	33
Have you collaborated with USIP staff or Fellows on projects since your Fellowship ended?	48%	67	48%	33

SOURCE: Survey of former Fellows; data tabulations by staff.

As Table 3-9 shows, the Fellows from more recent years are much less likely to have participated in any USIP events since their Fellowship ended. This might be because earlier Fellows simply had more time to participate, or the ways in which USIP tries to engage its Fellows have changed. This might also reflect changes in the size of the USIP staff and the relationship between the staff and Fellows. It should also be noted that many Fellows move away from the Washington area after their Fellowship ends. So, in that sense, these numbers are quite high, but it may also partially explain the number of Fellows participating in USIP events.

The survey then asked Fellows about their views about the Fellowship Program. The questions were built around the phrase "to what extent do you agree with the following statements." Focusing on responses of 4 or 5 (where 5 meant "completely agree"), the responding Fellows clearly felt (as shown in Figure 3-9) that the Fellowship was a very valuable experience (average = 4.8) and that the Fellowship was prestigious (average = 4.4). (The committee examines views of other peace and security experts on the issue of prestige in the next chapter.)

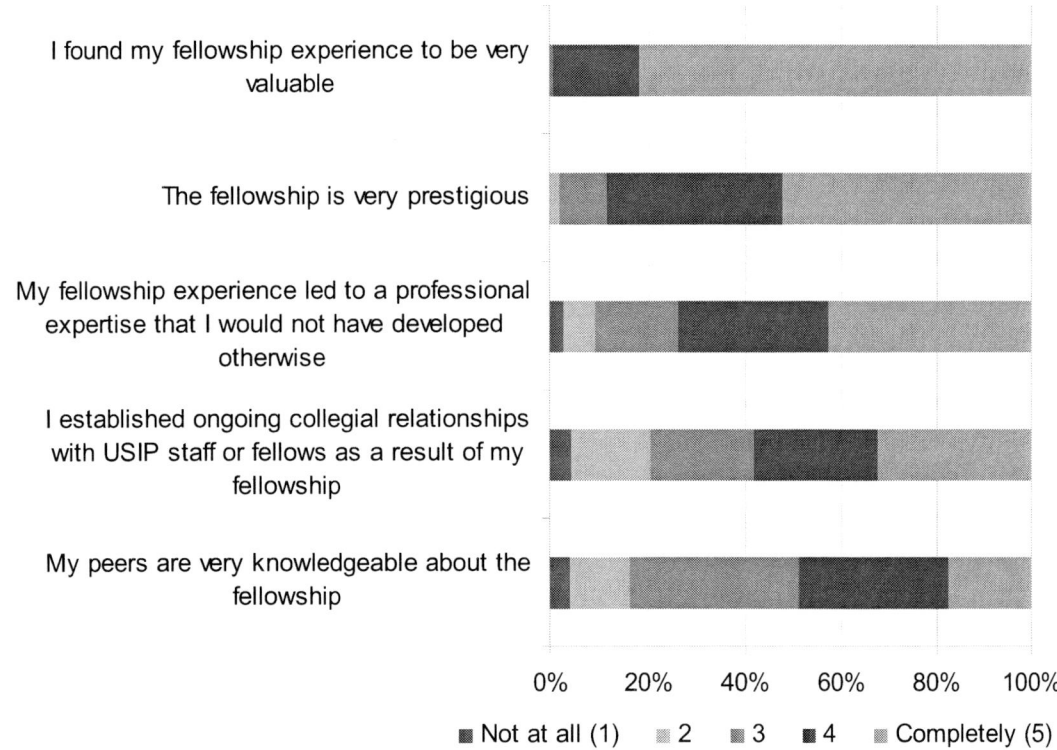

Figure 3-9 Percentage of respondents who agreed with various statements about the Fellowship
SOURCE: Survey of former Fellows; data tabulations by staff.
NOTE: Sample sizes differ slightly. They are, from top to bottom: 115, 113, 114, 114, and 113.

The areas where there was the lowest agreement concerned the establishment of ongoing collegial relationships with USIP staff or other Fellows (average = 3.7) and that Fellows' peers knew of the Fellowship (average = 3.5).

We then disaggregated those two factors by the period of the Fellowship (as shown in Table 3-10).

Table 3-10 Percentage of respondents, by period of Fellowship, who agreed with various statements about the Fellowship.

Comment	Fellows	Not at all (1)	2	3	4	Completely (5)	Hard to judge	Total
My peers are very knowledgeable about the Fellowship	1987-2001	3%	10%	34%	33%	16%	4%	70
	2002-2007	5%	15%	29%	22%	20%	10%	41
I established ongoing collegial relationships with USIP staff or fellows as a result of my fellowship	1987-2001	4%	24%	15%	23%	31%	3%	71
	2002-2007	5%	2%	29%	27%	32%	2%	41

SOURCE: Survey of former Fellows; data tabulations by staff.

There does not appear to be a significant difference between earlier and more recent Fellows on these two dimensions.

The survey then asked several questions regarding how helpful the Fellowship was to the Fellows. The scale ran from 1 to 5, where 5 meant "Very helpful." As Figure 3-10 illustrates, the largest effect—a goal of USIP—was to free up time for the Fellow to pursue his or her research.

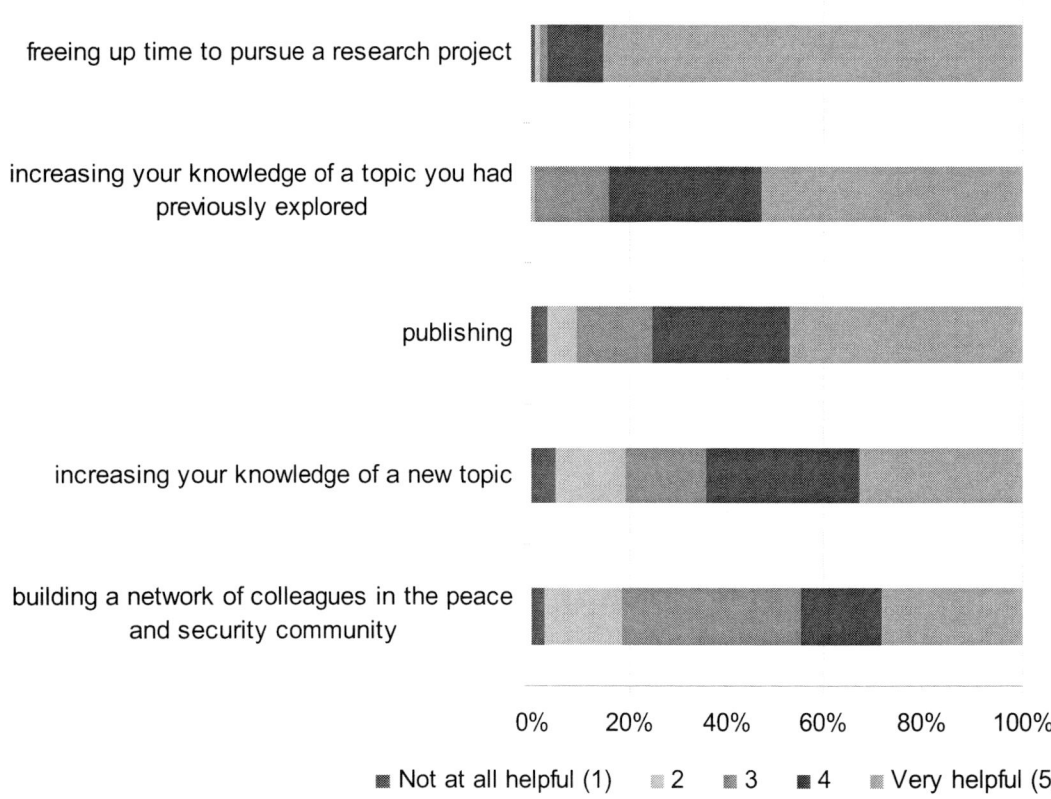

Figure 3-10 Percentage of respondents' saying the Fellowship was helpful in various ways
SOURCE: Survey of former Fellows; data tabulations by staff.
NOTE: n = 115, except for publishing (n = 112) and increasing knowledge of a new topic (n = 110).

The survey then focused more specifically on the question of networking by asking Fellows whether, as a result of the Fellowship, their networks were increased or not. As Figure 3-11 shows, respondents were most likely to report that their networks with the media tended to increase. In their relationships with others (e.g., government employees, nongovernmental (NGO) and intergovernmental organization representatives, and academics), about half of the Fellows reported that their contacts remained about the same while the other half reported that their contacts increased. While the Fellows tended to respond that their networks with academics stayed about the same, this may be because many Fellows are senior academics who already have large academic networks.

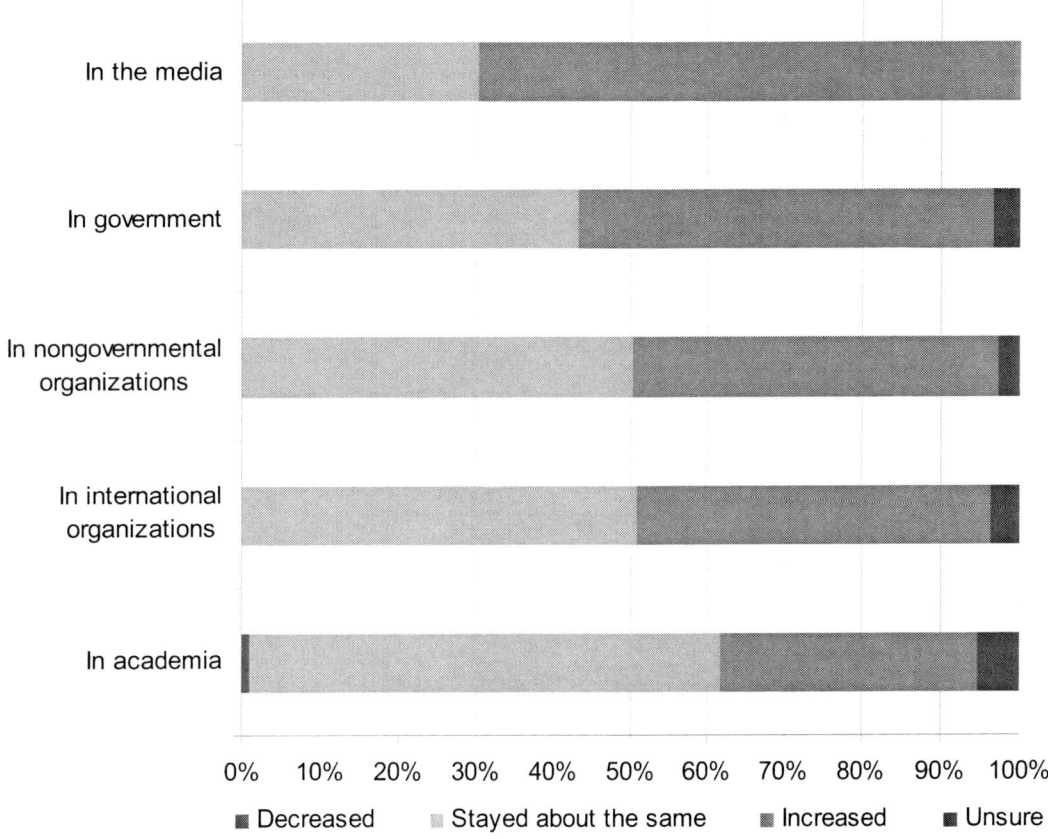

Figure 3-11 Changes to respondents' networks by type of actor
SOURCE: Survey of former Fellows; data tabulations by staff.
NOTE: Sample sizes differ slightly. They are from top to bottom: 112, 111, 113, 112, and 115.

These findings bear further study, since they may help USIP reach out to larger networks through the Fellows. Interviews or expert panels with Fellows to understand when a Fellow considers a person part of his or her "network," distinguishing colleagues from contacts, etc. could be helpful in this regard. Attention should be paid to the employment area from which the Fellow comes.

Next, the survey asked how satisfied Fellows were with various aspects of the Fellowship. The questions were scored on a scale from 1 to 5, where 1 was "Not at all satisfied" and 5 was "Extremely satisfied." Satisfaction was highest (a score of 5), as Figure 3-12 shows, for support from Fellowship staff, research assistant, and resources provided by USIP.

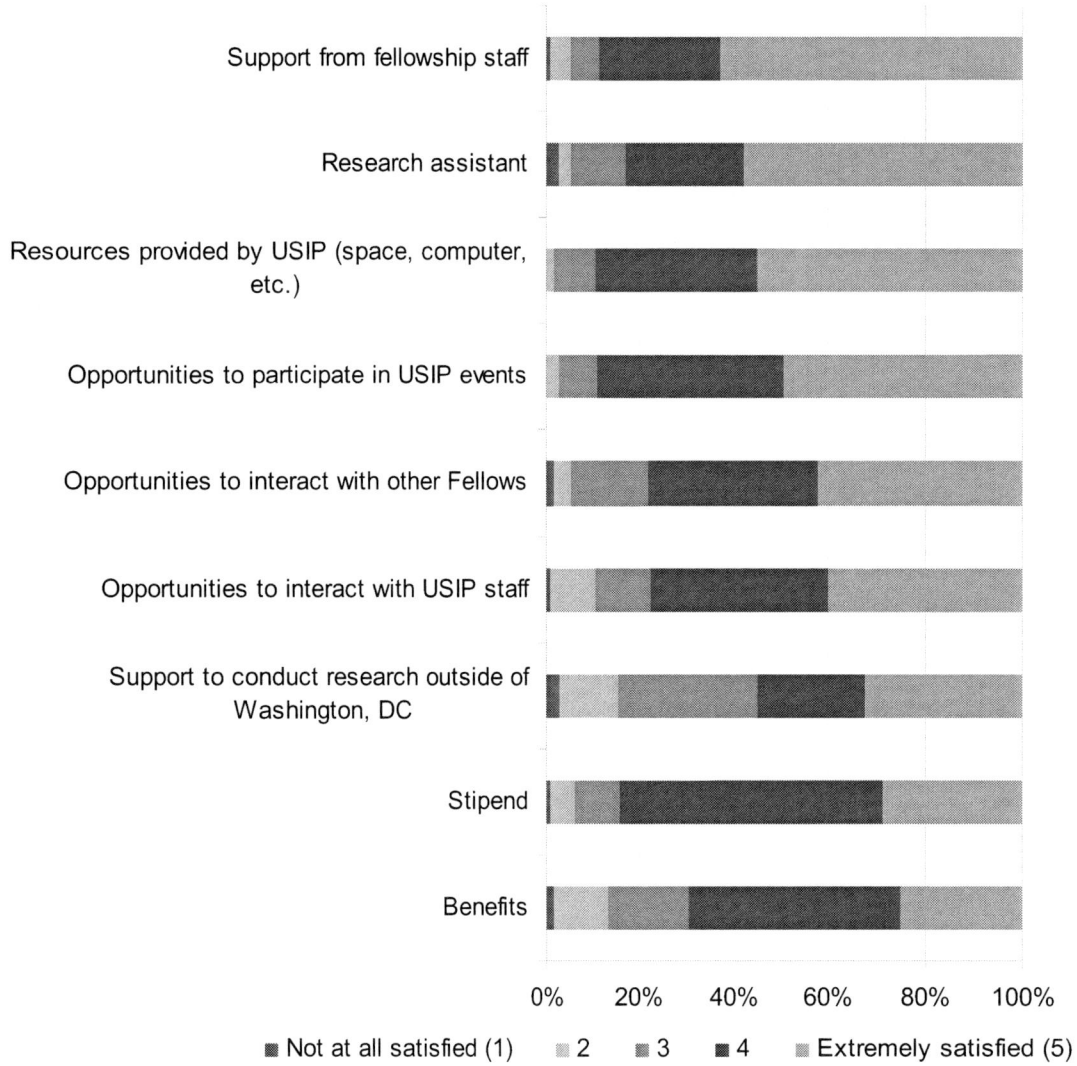

Figure 3-12 Respondents' degree of satisfaction with various characteristics of the Fellowship
SOURCE: Survey of former Fellows; data tabulations by staff.
NOTE: The sample size ranged between 111 and 115, except for support to conduct research outside of Washington, DC, which was answered by 105 of the 116 respondents.

Eighty percent of respondents reported that they were very satisfied or better (a score of 4 or 5) with each aspect of the program except for opportunities to interact with other fellows and USIP staff, support to conduct research outside of Washington, DC, and benefits. Improving the financial resources available to the Fellows may attract more and better applicants in the future. These findings suggest that some of the comments noted by respondents earlier in the chapter regarding the worst features of the program may have been the experiences of only a few respondents and are not shared among many former Fellows.

Finally, the survey asked the former Fellows whether they would recommend the Fellowship to others (Table 3-11) and then whether they had actually done so (Table 3-12).

Table 3-11 Whether respondents would recommend the Fellowship to others

Would you recommend the fellowship to others?	Percent
Yes	99
No	0
Don't know	1
Total	115

SOURCE: Survey of former Fellows; data tabulations by staff.

Table 3-12 Whether respondents have recommended the Fellowship to others

Have you recommended the fellowship to others?	Percent
Yes	96
No	2
Can't recall	2
Total	112

SOURCE: Survey of former Fellows; data tabulations by staff.

As both tables show, overwhelmingly the answer was yes.

To conclude the survey, a final question gave respondents the opportunity to raise any other issues or to comment on any aspect of the Fellowship. By and large, these comments continued the laudatory theme established in earlier responses.

> **"Probably one of the most fulfilling years of my professional life."**
>
> **"There is relatively little money available for research on conflict and peace issues, as the Jennings Randolph Program is perhaps the best known and most helpful program of support in this underfunded area available anywhere!"**
>
> **"A very successful program that provides excellent support to scholars who would like to take time off to pursue serious research. The program should continue."**
>
> **"It was a great opportunity."**
>
> **"The fellowship program is one of the central functions of USIP and is one of its greatest strengths."**

Fellows did have some suggestions for USIP; most common was a call for an alumni program:

> "I have often recommended that a more systematic effort be made by USIP to organize the alumni of the Fellows program. Universities do this well and the USG is attempting to build associate or reserve contingents. So far as I know, USIP does nothing to draw on the resources represented by alumni. Your questionnaire shows an interest in networking, and if that is one of your values, you should support a vigorous alumni program."

> "The USIP should be more proactive in maintaining links with its Fellows. The expertise of the Fellows is a resource which the USIP should continue to draw on for the work it does."

Additional suggestions included establishing complementary junior Fellowships, increasing resources, and improving mentoring/guidance.

> "While the Fellowship program targets and focuses on experts, USIP should consider expanding it to include providing more opportunities/Fellowships for people at more junior positions, e.g. someone at a mid point in their career, as opposed to well known scholars and experts."

> "The program needs to do a better job of promoting itself outside of the academic community. It needs to better publicize and promote the work of the fellows."

> "It is a wonderful program -- I only wish I were better able to take advantage of the opportunity from my end. If I were to recommend anything, it would be: 1) Give the [Jennings Randolph] program administrators a far larger budget to support Fellows for travel for the following purposes: research, field visits, conference presentations, etc. While I was able to scrape together enough funding from JR and other departments to do what I had hoped, it was not easy to pull off—and not possible for several of my JR colleagues, due to the lack of resources in this aspect of the JR program.... 2) Allow JR alumni to maintain their USIP email address for several years after their Fellowship, rather than just two months. 3) Allow a "free floating RA" to provide support for JR alumni once their Fellowships have ended -- because in many of our cases we need an RA after the Fellowship has ended even more than we do during the Fellowship."

> "Be more open from the outset as to the expectations that Fellows publish something as a result of the Fellowship. Establish some framework for structured interaction between the Fellows at the beginning, i.e. regular informal briefing sessions, because 9 months is too short a time for the Fellows to set this up themselves—it takes a

couple of months to realize it's not happening, by then there is a clear pattern of who is around the institute and who is not, and difficult at that stage to start anything."

FINDINGS

The survey of former Fellows, even considering the limitations cited earlier, suggests several findings:

1. A challenge for monitoring and evaluation is that a number of Fellows could not be located.

2. Fellows give the program high marks. A majority of fellows rated the program "excellent" (Figure 3-3, Table 3-5). Ninety-nine percent would recommend the fellowship to others, and 96 percent have actually done so (Tables 3-11, 3-12). Fellows overwhelmingly reported the experience to be very valuable (Figure 3-9). More than half of Fellows had their expectations completely met in five of eight criteria (Figure 3-4). The area where there was some concern, as was noted in some of the open-ended comments, lay in provision of resources to the Fellows. However, this point is somewhat contradicted later, when Fellows largely reported they were satisfied with resources provided by USIP (Figure 3-12). Overall there was a high degree of satisfaction with the various components of the program (Figure 3-12), and the program was seen as a boon to Fellows (Figure 3-5).

3. Fellows are very active in conducting research and disseminating information to multiple stakeholders. USIP gains a great deal from of the Fellows' time in Washington, DC. In terms of professional and career development activities, almost all Fellows were attending workshops, lectures, and seminars, and giving guest lectures. A majority were also advising or mentoring others (Figure 3-1, Table 3-2). Fellows were also involved in multiple forms of outreach as part of their Fellowship (Figure 3-2). A majority of Fellows conducted research in addition to their primary research project (Table 3-3), and about half or more of recent Fellows wrote op-eds, gave guest lectures, gave media interviews, or appeared on television or radio talk shows (Table 3-4).

4. Fellows have many opportunities to network with others and are generally satisfied with the amount of opportunities. Almost all Fellows found the Fellowship to be useful to increasing their network of colleagues (Figure 3-5). This was especially the case for networking with academics, but less so for government officials and the media (Figure 3-6). (Although building a network of colleagues was seen as the least useful of several functions of the

Fellowship (Figure 3-10). And while Fellows might not have seen the Fellowship as helpful in the case of media, it is noteworthy that about 70 percent of Fellows noted that their network with media increased (Figure 3-11).

5. Fellows tend to remain in contact with USIP and participate in USIP activities after the Fellowship ends. More than half of Fellows continued to stay in touch with USIP, participated in USIP events, and stayed in touch with other Fellows (Figure 3-8, Table 3-9).

6. Most Fellows reported ten months to be an appropriate duration for the Fellowship, although some thought that the Fellowship should be longer (Figure 3-7).

7. Finally, Fellows are unsure how well-known the Fellowship is, though they think the Fellowship is prestigious (Figure 3-9, Table 3-10). This point is further explored in the next chapter.

Chapter 4

Perceptions of the Peace and Security Community

Defining the external peace and security community is difficult. Nevertheless, it is important to identify it because the community is: (1) a source of future Fellows; (2) a consumer of Fellows' work (e.g., read publications, attend briefings); and (3) a source of potential research collaborators and participants in USIP activities. For these reasons at least, it is important to ascertain the views of this community toward USIP and its Fellows.

As noted in Chapter 1, the committee conducted a survey of a sample of peace and security experts, drawn from academia, nongovernmental/non-profit organizations (NGOs), and government. Sixty-five experts responded to the survey, most of whom were academics. Readers are cautioned against inferring the opinions of the respondents beyond this group to a larger community of experts. Rather, one should see the survey as a first step in examining how the Jennings Randolph Fellowships are viewed by those outside USIP. Nevertheless, some interesting findings are noted.

As a starting point, we wanted to see if experts were familiar with the USIP Fellowship Program. There was a concern that if the survey focused solely on the USIP Fellowship, topic interest or salience might be a factor: Individuals sent the survey might not respond if they thought that USIP fellowships were uninteresting to them. To combat this, the survey identified four senior fellowships: the Woodrow Wilson International Center for Scholars Fellowship program; the U.S. Department of State Franklin Fellowships program; the AAAS Science & Technology Policy Fellowships in National Defense & Global Security; and the U.S. Institute of Peace Jennings Randolph Senior Fellowships. (The USIP Fellowship was presented last for technical reasons: respondents not familiar with the program skipped to the end of the survey, since it made no sense to ask them specific questions about the Fellowship.) Box 4-1 provides summaries of the other three senior fellowships. The four programs share some similarities: applicants are senior experts; residency in Washington, DC; an approximately one year residency; a rigorous selection process. But there are also some differences: citizenship requirements; type of sponsor; target audience; and the number of years the program has been in existence).

Box 4-1
Descriptions of Senior Fellowships Programs

The Woodrow Wilson International Center for Scholars "supports research in the social sciences and humanities. Men and women from a wide variety of backgrounds, including government, the non-profit sector, the corporate world, and the professions, as well as academia, are eligible for appointment. Through an international competition, it offers nine-month residential fellowships to academics, public officials, journalists, and business professionals. Fellows conduct research and write in their areas of interest, while interacting with policymakers in Washington and Wilson Center staff. The Center also hosts Public Policy Scholars and Senior Scholars who conduct research and write in a variety of disciplines. In addition to the **Wilson Center Fellowships Program**, several of our regional programs have their own grant competitions (Africa, Asia, Canada, East Europe, Southeast Europe, Russia)."

"Since the end of the Cold War, the range and complexity of issues facing the international community has grown exponentially; the Department relies now on over 40 bureaus and offices to manage all aspects of bilateral and multilateral diplomacy. In order to strengthen its ability to deal with this plethora of issues and to draw on expertise of individuals working in disciplines related to them, the Department of State has launched the **'Franklin Fellows Program.'** This effort will provide unique opportunities for experienced professionals with a minimum of five years of relevant experience to spend a sabbatical year or detail as Fellows at the Department of State. The goal of the program is for Fellows, serving as consultants, to provide valuable and pertinent advice, views, opinions, alternatives or recommendations on foreign policy issues facing the nation."

"The American Association for the Advancement of Science manages and administers **Science & Technology Policy Fellowships** in six areas to provide the opportunity for accomplished scientists and engineers to participate in and contribute to the federal policymaking process while learning firsthand about the intersection of science and policy. The fellowships in congressional offices are funded by approximately 30 partner scientific and engineering societies. The fellowships in executive branch agencies are funded by the hosting offices. The fellowships are highly competitive and use a peer-review selection process. Review is followed by individual interviews in Washington, DC, conducted by selection committees comprised of professionals with expertise in the interface of science, technology, and policy. Following selection, Fellows come to Washington, DC, in September of each year and participate in a comprehensive orientation program before beginning their fellowships in the various sectors of government. AAAS also conducts a professional development program throughout the year. The fellowship programs have several basic requirements in common. Applicants must have a Ph.D. or an equivalent doctoral-level degree at the time of application. Individuals with a master's degree in engineering and at least three years of post-degree professional experience also may apply. Some programs require additional experience. Applicants must be U.S. citizens. Federal employees are not eligible for the fellowships."

Sources: Woodrow Wilson International Center for Scholars, available at http://www.wilsoncenter.org/index.cfm?fuseaction=sf.welcome; U.S. Department of State, Franklin Fellows Program (July 2008), available at http://www.careers.state.gov/docs/FF-Factsheet.pdf; and American Association for the Advancement of Science, available at http://fellowships.aaas.org/01_About/01_index.shtml.

The survey first asked about familiarity with these four programs. It is appropriate to consider respondents' answers within a program, but not necessarily between programs. In particular, the U.S. Department of State Franklin Fellows Program is quite new, and the AAAS program has a more limited target audience for potential fellows. These facts may explain the results immediately below. Table 4-1 considers respondents' familiarity with the programs.

Table 4-1 Familiarity with various senior peace and security fellowships

Fellowship Program	1 (Not at all familiar)	2	3	4	5 (Extremely familiar)
U.S. Institute of Peace Jennings Randolph Senior Fellowships	20%	16%	20%	23%	20%
Woodrow Wilson International Center for Scholars fellowship program	9%	23%	34%	20%	14%
U.S. Department of State Franklin fellowships program	71%	14%	9%	3%	3%
AAAS Science & Technology Policy Fellowships in National Defense & Global Security	54%	19%	14%	14%	0%

SOURCE: Survey of experts; data tabulations by staff.
NOTE: Based on 65 respondents, except for USIP results which were based on 64 respondents.

As the table shows, experts are more likely to be familiar with the Woodrow Wilson and USIP programs. Overall, familiarity with the USIP Fellowship is high (see Table 4-2), although one in five respondents was not at all familiar with the program.

Table 4-2 Mean familiarity with various senior peace and security fellowships

Fellowship Program	Mean
U.S. Institute of Peace Jennings Randolph Senior Fellowships	3.1
Woodrow Wilson International Center for Scholars fellowship program	3.1
AAAS Science & Technology Policy Fellowships in National Defense & Global Security	1.9
U.S. Department of State Franklin fellowships program	1.5

SOURCE: Survey of experts; data tabulations by staff.
NOTE: Based on 65 respondents, except for USIP results which were based on 64 respondents.

For those individuals who reported that they were not at all familiar with the USIP program, the survey ended at this point. For those that were familiar with the USIP program, the survey next asked respondents to rate the prestige of each of the four programs noted earlier. One concern was to take familiarity into account. This is because a respondent might report that they were not at all familiar with a program and then say that they thought it was extremely prestigious. To account for this possibility, the prestige scores were weighted by the respondents' response to familiarity. First, the responses of the respondents are presented in Table 4-3.

Table 4-3 Prestige of various senior peace and security fellowships

Fellowship Program	Degree of Prestige					
	1 (Not at all prestigious)	2	3	4	5 (Extremely prestigious)	Unsure
U.S. Institute of Peace Jennings Randolph Senior Fellowships	0%	0%	29%	46%	15%	10%
Woodrow Wilson International Center for Scholars fellowships	0%	0%	4%	52%	40%	4%
U.S. Department of State Franklin fellowships	0%	4%	10%	17%	2%	67%
AAAS Science & Technology Policy Fellowships in National Defense & Global Security	0%	0%	17%	31%	4%	48%

SOURCE: Survey of experts; data tabulations by staff.
NOTE: Based on 48 respondents.

Respondents ranked the Woodrow Wilson and USIP fellowships quite highly. In both cases, the modal response was 4 out of 5. The unweighted means were 3.8 for the USIP and AAAS fellowships, 4.4 for the Woodrow Wilson fellowships, and 3.5 for the U.S. Department of State fellowships. Respondents for the Woodrow Wilson and USIP fellowships were also more certain in their answers, as noted by the low percentage of respondents who selected "unsure" as an answer.

The next step was to weight prestige by familiarity. This was done by multiplying the respondent's familiarity score for each fellowship by the respective prestige score. This gives a new scale from 1 to 25.[1] The results are shown in Table 4-4.

---

[1] Note that the theoretical scale is from 1 to 25 for three fellowships and 2 to 25 for the USIP Fellowships, since anyone who responded with a 1 on familiarity would not have been given the option of answering the prestige question. A 2 would occur for a familiarity score of 2 (lowest possible) times a prestige score of 1 (lowest possible).

Table 4-4 Weighted prestige of various senior peace and security fellowships

Fellowship Program	Weighted Prestige Mean	S.D.
Woodrow Wilson International Center for Scholars fellowships	11.3	7.4
U.S. Department of State Franklin fellowships	8.4	5.2
AAAS Science & Technology Policy Fellowships in National Defense & Global Security	9.9	4.6
U.S. Institute of Peace Jennings Randolph Senior Fellowships	11.9	6.9

SOURCE: Survey of experts; data tabulations by staff.
NOTE: Excludes those who answered "unsure."

As the table shows, prestige was on the high end for the USIP Fellowship. It is important to note the limitations of this analysis. Respondents are likely thinking about the prestige of the program *currently*. There are also other historical fellowships that are not offered today. Over time, such organizations as the W. Alton Jones Foundation, the Ford Foundation, the MacArthur Foundation, the Social Science Research Council, among others, have offered programs in peace and security. It would be interesting to ask Fellows whether they had applied for other fellowships and how they rated USIP's program at the time compared with others in the field. A second approach would be to ask peace and security experts periodically how they rate the prestige of the USIP program, using the data collected here as a benchmark.

Next the survey asked experts if they knew any Fellows. As Table 4-5 shows, a wide majority did.

Table 4-5 Percentage of respondents who knew any USIP Jennings Randolph Senior Fellows

Respondent knows any USIP Jennings Randolph Senior Fellows?	Percent
Yes	64
No	24
Unsure	11
N	45

SOURCE: Survey of experts; data tabulations by staff.

At this point, the survey sought to tap the opinion of experts regarding their perceptions of the impact of the USIP Fellowship. Table 4-6 focuses on three possible impacts of the Fellowship: networking, increasing knowledge, and developing new tools.

Table 4-6 Respondents' views on importance of the Fellowships

How important do you think the Jennings Randolph Senior Fellowships are:	1 (Not at all important)	2	3	4	5 (Extremely important)	Unsure	N
In providing opportunities to bring people to Washington to network with experts in peace and security issues?	0%	2%	16%	38%	29%	16%	45
To increasing knowledge on peace and security topics, such as the nature of conflict or conflict resolution?	0%	7%	20%	30%	30%	14%	44
To developing new tools to manage, mitigate, or resolve conflicts?	2%	13%	29%	20%	18%	18%	45

SOURCE: Survey of experts; data tabulations by staff.

As the preceding table shows, in general, respondents thought the USIP Fellowship was important in all of these areas. The next question focused on the output of the Fellows themselves (see Table 4-7).

Table 4-7 Respondents' views on Fellows' output

Would you say that the Jennings Randolph Senior Fellows	1 (Not at all important)	2	3	4	5 (Extremely important)	Unsure	N
perform cutting-edge research?	4%	11%	36%	22%	4%	22%	45
support policymakers by providing analyses, policy options, or advice?	0%	13%	29%	31%	9%	18%	45

SOURCE: Survey of experts; data tabulations by staff.

As Table 4-7 shows, there was more disagreement over the degree to which USIP Fellows performed cutting-edge research. There was a more positive outlook on the role of the Fellows in supporting policymakers. A final question in this series then asked whether the return on investment matched up with the cost of the program.[2] Again, as Table 4-8 shows, there was a generally positive response. Additional research could shed light on what exactly was seen as the "return on investment."

Table 4-8 Respondents' views on return on investment of the program

Respondent reporting the return on investment that the USIP receives from the Jennings Randolph Senior Fellowship program is well worth the cost	Percentage
1 (Not at all)	0
2	2
3	22
4	31
5 (To a very great extent)	18
Unsure	27
Total	45

SOURCE: Survey of experts; data tabulations by staff.

The final question asked respondents if they had ever recommended to anyone that s/he should apply for the Fellowship program. A majority had not, as is shown in Table 4-9.

Table 4-9 Whether respondent has ever recommended to anyone that s/he should apply for the Fellowship

Respondent has ever recommended anyone apply to the fellowship program	Percent
Yes	39
No	59
Unsure	2
Total	44

SOURCE: Survey of experts; data tabulations by staff.

However, we do see a positive correlation ($r = 0.47$) between familiarity and whether a respondent had recommended the program to someone (as shown in Table 4-10). It seems that one would first need to be at least somewhat familiar with the program in order to recommend it to someone, although this might then feedback on degree of familiarity. Thus, steps to increase familiarity may also have a positive impact on applications.

---

[2] This question may be subject to measurement error since different respondents might have different opinions about what "return on investment" and "cost" mean.

Table 4-10 Relationship between familiarity and recommendation by respondent

Recommend anyone to be a Fellow?	Degree of familiarity				
	2	3	4	5	Total
Yes	0	3	5	9	17
No	7	7	8	4	26
Total	7	10	13	13	43

SOURCE: Survey of experts; data tabulations by staff.

The survey concluded with an open-ended question asking respondents if they had any additional comments that they would like to share with the committee.[3] Very few respondents wrote in anything, but there were a handful of interesting comments that are noteworthy.

1. General support for program:

"**The Jennings Randolph Fellowships are very valuable. They help scholars publish important work that often would never be written without Jennings Randolph support.**"

2. We got opposing views, suggesting more research is needed. For instance:

"**I think it is a great idea, but that there is all too often NOT the kind of theoretical work done that really could be framed as "cutting edge"—much if the time it is rather traditional poli sci or soc perspectives.**"

"**The policy-relevant research component of USIP through the JR program seems to have atrophied in recent years relative to USIP's emphasis on field activities in support of the USG and on DC networking functions.**"

3. Question of focus of USIP program—respondents are not sure what USIP's focus is.

"**Is this fellowship associated with the narrow definition of security issues or the wider one?**"

"**These are senior fellowships that go either to senior academics or those with first-hand experience in conflict zones around the world. I think Washington benefits from the latter fellows; I think the field of CR [conflict resolution] benefits more from the first category and I wish there were more of those, and fewer journalists, among USIP fellows over time.**"

---

[3] A final question was whether the respondent's employment sector was in academia, government, or nongovernmental/nonprofit organizations. The committee hoped to disaggregate the responses by type of employer, but there were too few responses from government employees to do this.

FINDINGS

Based solely on the respondents' answers, recognizing the substantial limitations of this very small survey, and reflecting the final part of the committee's charge, the committee draws five findings:

1. A wide majority of respondents (79 percent) had some familiarity with the USIP Fellowship Program (Table 4-1). More than two-thirds of respondents knew one or more Fellows (Table 4-5).
2. External commentators gave the Fellowship relatively high marks for prestige (Tables 4-3, 4-4). Sixty-one percent of respondents rated the program either a 4 or a 5, with a modal answer of 4.
3. Respondents reported that the Fellowship was seen to be important as a networking opportunity and to increase knowledge. There was less agreement on its importance to developing new tools to respond to conflict (Table 4-6).
4. The Fellows' role was seen by respondents as somewhat more important in supporting policymakers by providing information than in performing cutting edge research (Table 4-7).
5. Finally, while respondents were familiar with the program and many knew a Fellow, a majority had not recommended to anyone that s/he should apply for the Fellowship to anyone (Table 4-9).

Chapter 5

Recommendations for Next Steps

Since this is the first, formal evaluation of the Jennings Randolph Fellowship Program, the committee placed significant emphasis on providing advice to USIP for how to ensure that monitoring and evaluation become an established part of the program in the future. It also has a few recommendations, based on the survey of former Fellows, for steps that could improve the Fellowship itself. These recommendations are presented below, along with some supporting material where further explanation is needed to support and clarify the committee's suggestions.

Gathering Additional Data

USIP has accumulated a substantial amount of information about applicants and Fellows, but the committee also encountered some significant limitations. The spreadsheet created by USIP (data categories are presented in Table 1-2) is a useful tool for collecting and organizing data on the applicants and Fellows. The committee recommends that:

- USIP continue to collect the data for new applicants and fellows.
- USIP contact fellows to collect data currently missing from the spreadsheet.
- USIP collect new data to facilitate a better description of applicants and fellows. In particular, USIP could include a longer project description in the spreadsheet and could identify fellows as to whether they consider themselves to be scholars or practitioners.

Understanding How Fellows' Research Advances USIP and U.S. Foreign Policy Goals

For a number of reasons discussed earlier in the report, the committee was not able to make much progress in meeting this part of its charge beyond presenting a basic overview of Fellows' research. To complete the second part of the committee's charge and to better interpret the findings above, the committee recommends the following strategy:

- USIP should conduct interviews or expert panels with former and current staff and board members to trace and assess the evolution of USIP's goals with respect both to the Fellowship program and the USIP mandate.
- USIP may wish to take a similar approach and collect information from external actors (e.g., government officials, academic experts, etc.). Although, ultimately, the program should be evaluated based on USIP's rationale, it would nevertheless be interesting to see how these actors judged the purpose of the fellowship. (A start at

this approach is that both the survey of Fellows and the survey of peace and security experts included questions on this, as presented in Chapters 3 and 4.)

- <u>USIP should take steps to identify U.S. foreign policy goals to see how the working of the program relates to broader U.S. foreign policy goals.</u>

    The committee suggests that a strategy for accomplishing this would involve identifying important foreign policy challenges or goals and examining which of those areas Fellows are researching—both before and after these challenges or goals are identified by policymakers and other "thought leaders." This would enable USIP to begin to examine whether the research done under its aegis lags or leads larger policy issues.

    There are a number of ways to describe changes in U.S. foreign policy goals from 1987 to the present. There is no single authoritative source of information about U.S. foreign policy goals on which USIP could rely. If, as a government-funded institution, USIP's primary concern is with official goals, then one could make use of the statements of foreign and security policy strategies that the White House has issued under most recent presidents. These are not always updated annually, but they do represent the product of an extensive interagency process. One could also undertake a content analysis of key speeches by government leaders, which would offer the option of including the views of Congress.

    If one wanted to move beyond official documents, an analysis of frequently cited terms in media reports would offer another way to track changes in goals over time. Survey data could offer the perceptions of foreign policy elites inside and out of government; an example of this is the series of surveys, "American Public Opinion and Foreign Policy," conducted by the Chicago Council on Foreign Relations every four years since 1978 (CCFR 2004). The survey results could be employed to create a framework for comparing applicants and Fellow's research to broader foreign policy concerns. The surveys involve both interviews of leaders and a survey of public opinion; it is the elite opinions that are relevant here. Leaders "with foreign policy power, specialization, and expertise" include "Congressional members or their senior staff, university administrators and academics who teach in the area of international relations, journalists and editorial staff who handle international news, administration officials and other senior staff in various agencies and offices dealing with foreign policy, religious leaders, senior business executives from FORTUNE 1,000 corporations, labor presidents of the largest labor unions, presidents of major private foreign policy organizations, and presidents of major special interest groups relevant to foreign policy (CCFR 2005)." The relevant survey question for the committee's purposes is: "What do you feel are the two or three biggest foreign policy problems facing the United States today?" Over the course of surveys from 1978-2002, 67 different problems were identified. The top five issues for each survey from 1986 through 2002 are summarized in Table 5-1; the complete list may be found in Appendix D. The next step would be to examine the body of work produced by Fellows in the three years prior to and after each survey. This would be most efficiently done by surveying each Fellow and asking which of the problems identified s/he thought his or her work focused on (and perhaps the most important problem). This may be a more elaborate effort than USIP would want to undertake; the example is offered to suggest that there are a variety of ways in which USIP could assess U.S. foreign policy goals that could be relevant to the Fellowship.

Table 5-1 Top 5 foreign policy problems identified in Chicago Council on Foreign Relations surveys, 1986-2002

1986	Russia/dealings with Russia (46 percent); Arms Control (33 percent); Latin/South/Central America (28 percent); Balance of Payments (17 percent); Mid-East Situation (Non-specific) (11 percent); Terrorism (11 percent)
1990	Iraq (Saddam Hussein (44 percent); Mid-East Situation (non-specific) (29 percent); Russia/dealings with Russia (21 percent); International Trade (18 percent); World Economy (14 percent)
1994	International Trade (24 percent); Russia/dealings with Russia (23 percent); Weak leadership (19 percent); Stronger U.S. Foreign Policy Needed (16 percent); Our Relationship with Bosnia (16 percent)
1998	World Economy (21 percent); Iraq (Saddam Hussein) (18 percent); Arms Control (15 percent); Russia/dealing with Russia (13 percent); Japan/Asian Economy/Crisis (13 percent)
2002	Terrorism (50 percent); Mid-East Situation (non-specific) (38 percent); Unrest in Israel/Israel-Palestine (16 percent); India and Pakistan Issues (14 percent); Arms Control (9 percent)

The survey findings also raise an issue about the purpose of the fellowship that could be further explored. Specifically, <u>USIP should investigate whether to seek Fellows to advance thinking and offer more cutting-edge thinking in targeted areas, or focus on the application of such thinking to USIP priority issues.</u>

Making Monitoring and Evaluation a Regular Part of the Fellowship
<u>The committee feels strongly that USIP should undertake more rigorous and systematic monitoring and evaluation (M&E) of the Fellowship in the future</u>. There are a number of approaches that USIP could take to develop a useful M&E strategy:
- Conduct an evaluation midway through the Fellowship to assess the match between resources and the Fellow's productivity, and to ascertain whether flexibility in timing and travel is needed.
- Hold an exit interview with all Fellows at the conclusion of the Fellowship. An interview could focus on such topics as:
    1. identify the various activities that Fellows pursued and how much time they spent on them.
    2. a list of Fellows' output, in particular asking what the Fellows believe to be their most important work. This could be done by collecting Fellow's CVs.
- Conduct an impact assessment of Fellows' work, completed during their Fellowship period. Ideally, such an approach would consist of (1) identifying all the products a Fellow produced during or directly related to the Fellowship, and (2) quantifying the impact of those works.

In practice, the ideal is unlikely to be met. Fellows' communications with others, briefings, and other informal interactions may inspire others, lead to policies, spur research, etc. It is very difficult to ascertain the impact of a Fellow's briefing of Congressional staff member, for instance. However, as noted above, many Fellows who responded to the survey reported that a written work was their most important contribution and this is a good area to start and one that can be quantified. Three different measures will serve to illustrate possible approaches. Scopus and Google Scholar both count citations to authors' work,[1] while Web hits (using the Fellow's name and title of publication as search terms) could also be examined. Related to this strategy, one could also look at where Fellows publish, in particular, which of their products were published by USIP Press, and which works funded by the fellowship were published in "top" academic presses or "top" journals in the field. A CV analysis would be helpful to this end.

- Conduct an impact assessment of the Fellowship on Fellows' careers. Once an initial assessment was undertaken, the process could be updated on a periodic basis.

There are a number of possible directions that USIP might pursue. Since these are senior fellowships, the spotlight could be on Fellows' research or their collaborations with other peace and security experts—in both cases comparing the time before and after the Fellowship, rather than focusing on their employment. That said, it might also be instructive to ask former Fellows how the Fellowship helped them advance in their careers (e.g., for academics, did the Fellowship have a positive impact on their receiving tenure or a promotion). Two methodologies for collecting this information are collecting CVs of Fellows or via a survey. The survey approach is more efficient in that one could ask Fellows what work before and after their Fellowship they consider to be related to their work at USIP. One could also survey Fellows to get a sense of how they view the research they conducted during the Fellowship: as a unique project, or as the beginning or the culmination of a research agenda. The latter could be done via a social network analysis. Social network analysis maps the relationships between individuals in networking or collaborative activities. One purpose of the analysis could be to test the hypothesis that the Fellowships increase Fellows' networks; another could be to examine in more detail the groups of people Fellows' interact with (e.g. academics, practitioners, media, or government officials).

In implementing any of the suggestions for its approach to M&E provided above, it would be worthwhile to further disaggregate the Fellows into demographic categories to see if different groups of Fellows have significantly different views or outcomes. One category would be U.S. versus foreign Fellows. Although this is a "senior" fellowship, it might be possible to differentiate between more junior and senior individuals within this aforementioned group. A third category would be the Fellows' employment sector (e.g., academia, media, etc.).

---

[1] An alternative to Scopus is ISI's Web of Science.

Understanding External Perceptions of the Fellowship

The committee also makes several recommendations intended to help USIP gain further knowledge about the perceptions of the Fellowships in the wider expert community.

- USIP should continue to probe the external peace and security community about their perceptions of the program's impact. Information collected can assist USIP in reaching out to a broader audience, better tailoring its message, and improving competition for the fellowship by increasing the number of qualified applicants.
  1. Information collected should include topics from the survey of experts. Additional topics might include whether peace and security experts had collaborated on research or other projects with Fellows; whether they used work produced by Fellows in their research, teaching, or practice; or particular Fellows' products that experts thought were especially useful or influential.
  2. Information should be collected from a broad range of experts, including academics, nongovernmental/nonprofit organization employees, and government employees.

     The committee's survey focused on academics at peace and conflict centers. Many more academics would be included in the relevant population. USIP may wish to partner with relevant professional associations or seek to develop its own list of relevant academics. An important point is that for much of this information to be useful, USIP needs to pre-identify individuals for inclusion in any future surveys those who have some familiarity with the program. Such a list could start, but must go beyond, participants in USIP events and activities. Likewise the survey focused on representatives of NGOs with a focus on peace and conflict. One could also look to NGOs with a regional focus first, who work on conflict issues as a subtheme.

- USIP should consider mixed modes to collect the data, reflecting the challenges of tapping different types of respondents' views.

  Getting in touch with government employees proved the most difficult, and they were least likely to answer the survey. Future efforts to reach government employees would be better accomplished through expert panels or face-to-face interviews. This is facilitated by the fact that USIP staff and government employees are co-located in Washington, DC. It should be noted that for some potential respondents, confidentiality could be an issue. Again, USIP needs to pre-identify individuals who have some familiarity with the program. Academics responded well to a survey, so it may be worthwhile to conduct a more targeted survey to a broader range of academics, assuming a better population can be identified. Academics can also be reached for expert panels or interviews at major conferences or at other venues. NGO employees are, like academics, spread throughout the nation, and so they may best be reached via a survey. However, they may require more follow-ups than the academics do to ensure an adequate response rate.

- USIP's future research on the views of the expert community should seek more in-depth commentary on the impact of the program.

  The committee asked a question on familiarity. A logical follow-up is to probe more into how experts hear about the program and their connections to the

Fellowship (e.g., attending Fellows' briefings, reading Fellows' reports, etc.). The committee asked a question on prestige. Follow-up questions might focus on what makes the Fellowship prestigious. What is it about fellows or their work that stands out? The committee did not ask about issues of balance or priorities, although it received some open-ended comments. One comment that was noted earlier had to do with appropriate balance between scholars and practitioners (to the extent that there is a divide between them). Related to this is the notion of what type of people should be Fellows (e.g., from which disciplines). Finally, future research could explore experts' views on what regions or topics USIP fellows ought to be covering. Such research could provide valuable information on how the direction of USIP matches the perceptions of the external community.

Improving the Fellowship Experience

Based on the survey results, the Committee recommends certain steps be considered to improve the Fellowship:

- Explore setting up an alumni network for former Fellows. Such a network could take advantage of the current USIP website or involve a new product, for example by tapping a social network site. One way to facilitate a network would be to hold a meeting of Fellows designed to build such a network.
- Consider establishing support from businesses or associations in the community to help fellows and families cope with expenses of life in the D.C. area.
- Consider the potential for and ramifications of allowing for extensions of time to the Fellowship in individual cases. Some fellows and USIP may benefit greatly from having individual fellowships extended for a few months. In addition, USIP might want to consider greater flexibility in travel and support options for research outside DC, especially internationally, during the Fellowship.

Bibliography

Boulding, E. 1992. Peace Research and the US Institute of Peace. *Peace Review* 4(1):46-50.

CCFR (Chicago Council on Foreign Relations). 2005. GLOBAL VIEWS 2004: AMERICAN
PUBLIC OPINION AND FOREIGN POLICY [Computer file]. ICPSR version. Menlo Park, CA: Knowledge Networks, Inc. [producer], 2004. Ann Arbor, MI: Inter-university Consortium for Political and Social Research [distributor].

CCFR (Chicago Council on Foreign Relations). 2004. AMERICAN PUBLIC OPINION AND U.S. FOREIGN POLICY, 2002 [Computer file]. ICPSR version. Rochester, NY: Harris Interactive [producer], 2002. Ann Arbor, MI: Inter-university Consortium for Political and Social Research [distributor].

Cohn, P. 2003. Peace at What Price? *Congress Daily* (October 31):12-13

Crocker, C. 2004. The Growth of a Unique Federal Agency: Reflections on the Past and Thoughts about the Future of the United States Institute of Peace. Washington, DC: USIP. Available at www.usip.org/events/2004/0804_transcrocker.html.

Montgomery, M.E. 2003. Working for Peace While Preparing for War: The Creation of the United States Institute of Peace. *Journal of Peace Research* 40(4):479-496.

Weigel, G. 1984/85. The United States Institute of Peace: From Contention to Contribution. *World Affairs* 147(3):191-200.

Wong, J. 1993. Institute of Peace, a Cold-War Creation, Charts New Course. The *Chronicle of Higher Education* 40(4):A30.

Appendix A
Committee Members

Major General William F. Burns (United States Army, Retired), *Chair*, was director of the Arms Control and Disarmament Agency from 1988 to 1989. He served as the first U.S. special envoy to denuclearization negotiations with former Soviet countries under legislation sponsored by former Sen. Sam Nunn (D-GA) and Sen. Richard Lugar (R-Ind.). He is a distinguished fellow at the Army War College. He is also an Arms Control Association board member.

Dr. Burt S. Barnow is associate director for research and principal research scientist at the Institute for Policy Studies of the Johns Hopkins University. Dr. Barnow received a B.S. in economics from the Massachusetts Institute of Technology and a Ph.D. in economics from the University of Wisconsin at Madison. His work focuses on the operation of labor markets and evaluating social programs, and his current research includes an evaluation of the welfare-to-work program, an evaluation of training programs to train U.S. workers for jobs currently filled with foreign workers who come to the United States on an H-1B visa, and an evaluation of New Hampshire's welfare reforms. Dr. Barnow also teaches program evaluation in the institute's graduate public policy program and labor economics in the Department of Economics. Before coming to Johns Hopkins, he was vice president of a consulting firm in the Washington, DC area. Dr. Barnow served nine years in the Department of Labor, most recently as director of the Office of Research and Evaluation for the Employment and Training Administration. Dr. Barnow recently co-chaired the NRC Committee on Workforce Needs in Information Technology.

Ms. Joyce Davis is currently senior vice president of WITF, Inc. in Harrisburg, PA. Prior to that, she worked in Prague as the associate director of broadcasting for Radio Free Europe/Radio Liberty. She is the former deputy foreign editor for Knight Ridder Newspapers. Prior to her work at Knight Ridder, Ms. Davis served as foreign editor and director of news staffing at National Public Radio, as well as an on-air reporter, doing special reports on the Middle East and the Palestinian-Israeli conflict. In her more than 30 years of journalism, Ms. Davis has been a reporter, columnist and editor in both broadcast and print. She began her journalism career at *The New Orleans Times-Picayune*. In 1997, Ms. Davis wrote *Between Jihad and Salaam: Profiles in Islam*, a collection of profiles and interviews with Islamic leaders around the world, which was published in 1997. Her most recent book is *Martyrs: Innocence, Vengeance and Despair in the Middle East*. Ms. Davis is a former Senior Fellow with the United States Institute of Peace, as well as a member of the Advisory Council of Women in International Security and the Georgetown University *Journal of International Affairs*.

Dr. Johanna Mendelson Forman is a senior associate at the Center for Strategic and International Studies (CSIS), where she works on the Americas, civil-military relations, and post-conflict reconstruction. A former codirector of the Post-Conflict Reconstruction Project, she has written extensively on security-sector reform in conflict states, economic development in postwar societies, and the role of the United Nations in peace operations.

In 2003, she participated in a review of the post-conflict reconstruction effort of the Coalition Provisional Authority in Iraq as part of a CSIS team. Dr. Mendelson Forman also brings experience in the world of philanthropy, having served as the director of peace, security, and human rights at the UN Foundation. She has held senior positions in the U.S. government at the U.S. Agency for International Development in the Bureau for Humanitarian Response and the Office of Transition Initiatives, as well as at the World Bank's Post Conflict Unit. She has been a senior fellow with the Association of the United States Army and a guest scholar at the U.S. Institute of Peace. Most recently, she served as an adviser to the UN Mission in Haiti. She holds adjunct faculty appointments at American University and Georgetown University. Dr. Mendelson Forman is a member of the Council on Foreign Relations and serves on the Advisory Council of Women in International Security and the advisory board of the Latin American Security Network, RESDAL. She holds a J.D. from Washington College of Law at American University, a Ph.D. in Latin American history from Washington University, St. Louis, and a master's of international affairs, with a certificate of Latin America studies, from Columbia University in New York.

Dr. P. Terrence Hopmann is professor of International Relations and director of the Conflict Management Program at The Paul H. Nitze School of Advanced International Studies of Johns Hopkins University, Washington, DC, and professor emeritus of Political Science, Brown University, Providence, RI. He specializes in the field of international security, negotiation, and conflict resolution. Dr. Hopmann received his B.A. from Princeton University's Woodrow Wilson School of Public and International Affairs and his M.A. and Ph.D. in Political Science from Stanford University. From 1968 through 1985, he served in the Political Science Department at the University of Minnesota, where he also directed the Quigley Center of International Studies and later the Stassen Center for World Peace in the Hubert H. Humphrey Institute of Public Affairs. At Brown he established the International Relations Program in 1986, and then became director of the Center for Foreign Policy Development in 1993, which later became the Global Security Program in the Thomas J. Watson Jr. Institute for International Studies, which he directed until 2004. After returning from a sabbatical leave in Washington, DC and Vienna, Austria in academic year 2004-05, he was appointed chair of Brown's Political Science Department. He has held numerous fellowships, including at the Woodrow Wilson International Center for Scholars, the Carnegie Endowment for International Peace, and the U.S. Institute of Peace, and through the Fulbright Program. He served from 1984-92 as a frequent consultant to the United Nations Development Programme and the UN Economic Commission for Latin America and the Caribbean, to the Foreign Ministries of Mexico and Brazil, and to the United Nations University for Peace in Costa Rica, which included the presentation of workshops on international negotiations for diplomats from throughout Latin America. He has also worked with USIP"s Training Program, participating in workshops on negotiation, conflict resolution, and regional security institutions in Budapest, Bangkok, and Bucharest. Dr. Hopmann has also developed and managed an on-line training course for U.S. volunteers with the OSCE maintained by USIP for the Department of State.

Dr. Kathryn Newcomer is a professor at the Trachtenberg School of Public Policy and Public Administration at the George Washington University where she is also codirector of the Midge Smith Center for Evaluation Effectiveness, home of The Evaluators' Institute, and she is the director of the Ph.D. in Public Policy and Administration program, and associate director of the School. She teaches public and nonprofit program evaluation, research design, and applied statistics. She routinely conducts research and training for federal and local government agencies and nonprofit organizations on performance measurement and program evaluation, and she has designed and conducted evaluations for several U.S. federal agencies and dozens of nonprofit organizations. Dr. Newcomer has published five books: *Improving Government Performance* (1989), *The Handbook of Practical Program Evaluation* (1994, 2nd edition 2004), *Meeting the Challenges of Performance-Oriented Government* (2002), *Getting Results: A Guide for Federal Leaders and Managers* (2005), and *Transforming Public and Nonprofit Organizations: Stewardship for Leading Change* (2008)—as well as a volume of *New Directions for Public Program Evaluation, Using Performance Measurement to Improve Public and Nonprofit Programs* (1997), and numerous articles in journals, among them the *Public Administration Review*. She is a Fellow of the National Academy of Public Administration, and currently serves on the Comptroller General's Educators' Advisory Panel. She served as president of the National Association of Schools of Public Affairs and Administration (NASPAA) for 2006-2007. She has received two Fulbright awards, one for Taiwan (1993) and one for Egypt (2001-04). She has lectured on performance measurement and public program evaluation in Ukraine, Brazil, Egypt, Taiwan, and the United Kingdom. Dr. Newcomer earned a B.S. in education and an M.A. in Political Science from the University of Kansas, and her Ph.D. in political science from the University of Iowa.

Dr. Karin von Hippel is codirector of the Center for Strategic and International Studies (CSIS) Post-Conflict Reconstruction Project and senior fellow with the CSIS International Security Program. Previously, she was a senior research fellow at the Centre for Defence Studies, King's College London, and spent several years working for the United Nations and the European Union in Somalia and Kosovo. In 2004 and 2005, she participated in two major studies for the UN: one on UN peacekeeping and the second on the UN humanitarian system. Also in 2004, she was part of a small team funded by the U.S. Agency for International Development to investigate the development potential of Somali remittances. In 2002, she advised the Organization for Economic Cooperation and Development on the role of development cooperation in discovering the root causes of terrorism. Since then, she has participated in numerous conferences and working groups on the subject in Africa, Europe, and North America. She also directed a project funded by the MacArthur Foundation on European counterterrorist reforms and edited the volume *Europe Confronts Terrorism* (Palgrave Macmillan 2005). She was a member of Project Unicorn, a counterterrorism police advisory panel in London. Additional publications include *Democracy by Force* (Cambridge 2000), which was short-listed for the Westminster Medal in Military History; "Report on Integrated Missions: Practical Perspectives and Recommendations" (UN ECHA Core Group 2005); "Counter Radicalization Development Assistance" (Danish Institute for International Studies 2006); and "Blurring of Mandates in Somalia" in *Humanitarian Diplomacy: Practitioners* *and Their Craft* (UN University Press 2007). She received her Ph.D. in international relations from the London School of Economics, her M.St. from Oxford University, and her B.A. from Yale University.

Dr. Christine Wing is senior fellow and project coordinator, Strengthening Multilateral Approaches to Nuclear and Biological Weapons, at the Center on International Cooperation, New York University. Her areas of expertise include: multilateral approaches to nuclear, biological and chemical weapons issues; U.S.-China and East Asian security issues; U.S. foreign and military policy; the role of NGOs in shaping foreign policies; and she has a geographical focus on China and East Asia. From 1995 to 2004, Dr. Wing was program officer for International Peace and Security at the Ford Foundation in New York. In that role she oversaw the foundation's funding concerned with weapons of mass destruction, the emerging security environment, and intrastate and regional conflict; she worked extensively with organizations in China and West Africa, as well in the United States. She has also served as a consultant to the Nuclear Threat Initiative, and was visiting fellow at Princeton University's Center of International Studies. From 1984-1989, Dr. Wing was also coordinator of the National Disarmament Program at the American Friends Service Committee (AFSC); and from 1979-1984 she was AFSC's National Representative for Economic Rights. She holds a Ph.D. in international security studies from the Woodrow Wilson School at Princeton University.

Dr. I. William Zartman is the Jacob Blaustein Professor of International Organizations and Conflict Resolution and director of the Conflict Management Program at The Paul H. Nitze School of Advanced International Studies (SAIS) of Johns Hopkins University. His areas of interest include: conflict resolution and negotiation; crisis management; developing nations; diplomacy; human rights; international relations; political risk analysis; treaty negotiations. Dr. Zartman was the former director of SAIS African Studies Program; former faculty member at the University of South Carolina and New York University; served as Olin Professor at the U.S. Naval Academy, Halevy Professor at the Institute of Political Studies in Paris, and visiting professor at the American University in Paris; was a consultant to the U.S. Department of State; was president of the Tangier American Legation Museum Society; and is past president of the Middle East Studies Association and the American Institute for Maghrib Studies. He holds a Ph.D. in international relations from Yale University.

Appendix B
Survey of Former Fellows

1. Survey of United States Institute of Peace Jennings Randolph Fellows

1. In what year did your fellowship begin?

Year _____

2. During your fellowship, did you engage in any of the following professional or career development activities (check all that apply)?

- [ ] Gave guest lectures
- [ ] Advised or mentored others
- [ ] Organized seminars or workshops
- [ ] Attended workshops, lectures, seminars in your research area

Other
_____

3. During your fellowship, which of the following activities did you engage in (check all that apply)?

- [ ] Conducted research aside from proposed research project
- [ ] Wrote op-ed(s) for newspapers
- [ ] Wrote article(s) for refereed journals
- [ ] Wrote article(s) for other journals or magazines
- [ ] Wrote special report(s)
- [ ] Wrote book manuscript(s)
- [ ] Wrote book chapter manuscript(s)
- [ ] Gave guest lecture(s)
- [ ] Gave media interviews
- [ ] Appeared on TV or radio talk shows
- [ ] Participated in congressional briefing(s)
- [ ] Gave congressional testimony
- [ ] Informally advised US government agencies

Other (please specify)
_____

4. How would rate the quality of the fellowship program overall

- ○ Poor (1)
- ○ 2
- ○ 3
- ○ 4
- ○ Excellent (5)

5. What do you think was the most important product you produced during your fellowship?

[text box]

6. Did the fellowship meet your expectations in...

	Not at all (1)	2	3	4	Completely (5)	Hard to judge
ability to conduct your own research	○	○	○	○	○	○
access to research facilitites and resources	○	○	○	○	○	○
ability to collaborate with others at USIP	○	○	○	○	○	○
ability to collaborate with others outside USIP	○	○	○	○	○	○
mentoring or advising	○	○	○	○	○	○
ability to publish your research	○	○	○	○	○	○
ability to attend conferences, meetings, etc.	○	○	○	○	○	○
administrative support from USIP	○	○	○	○	○	○

7. How useful was your fellowship in...

	Not at all useful (1)	2	3	4	Very useful (5)	Hard to judge
Increasing your knowledge of your fellowship research project	○	○	○	○	○	○
Improving research skills or techniques	○	○	○	○	○	○
Increase your opportunities to publish research	○	○	○	○	○	○
Increasing your network of colleagues	○	○	○	○	○	○

Other
[text box]

8. To what extent did you fellowship provide you with the opportunity to interact with the peace and security community?

	Not at all (1)	2	3	4	A great deal (5)	Hard to judge
Practitioners	○	○	○	○	○	○
Government officials	○	○	○	○	○	○
Members of international organizations	○	○	○	○	○	○
Members of non-profit or non-governmental oragnizations	○	○	○	○	○	○
Academics	○	○	○	○	○	○
Media	○	○	○	○	○	○

Other
[text box]

9. Is 10 months the right duration for the Fellowship?

○ Yes
○ No
○ Unsure

If no, how long do you think the Fellowship should be?
[text box]

10. What was the best feature of the fellowship?

[text box]

11. What was the worst feature of the fellowship?

[text box]

12. In what ways do you think the work you did during your fellowship was helpful to USIP?

[text box]

13. Do you continue to conduct research or work in the areas that your research project focused on?

- ◯ Yes
- ◯ No
- ◯ Not applicable

14. Have you continued to stay in touch with USIP staff or programs since your fellowship ended?

- ◯ Yes
- ◯ No
- ◯ Not applicable

15. Have you continued to stay in touch with any Jennings Randolph Fellows since your fellowship ended?

- ◯ Yes
- ◯ No
- ◯ Not applicable

16. Have you participated in any USIP events since your fellowship ended?

- ◯ Yes
- ◯ No
- ◯ Not applicable

If yes, about how many?

17. Have you collaborated with USIP staff or fellows on projects since your fellowship ended?

○ Yes
○ No
○ Not applicable

if yes, about how many projects?
_____

18. To what extent do you agree with the following statements:

	Not at all (1)	2	3	4	Completely (5)	Hard to judge
I found my fellowship experience to be very valuable	○	○	○	○	○	○
My fellowship experience led to a professional expertise that I would not have developed otherwise	○	○	○	○	○	○
The fellowship is very prestigious	○	○	○	○	○	○
My peers are very knowledgeable about the fellowship	○	○	○	○	○	○
I established ongoing collegial relationships with USIP staff or fellows as a result of my fellowship	○	○	○	○	○	○

19. Was the fellowship helpful in...

	Not at all helpful (1)	2	3	4	Very helpful (5)	Hard to judge
building a network of colleagues in the peace and security community	○	○	○	○	○	○
freeing up time to pursue a research project	○	○	○	○	○	○
publishing	○	○	○	○	○	○
increasing your knowledge of a topic you had previously explored	○	○	○	○	○	○
increasing your knowledge of a new topic	○	○	○	○	○	○

Other (please specify)
_____

20. As a result of your fellowship, would you say your network of colleagues increased, stayed about the same, or decreased?

	Decreased	Stayed about the same	Increased	Unsure
In academia	○	○	○	○
In government	○	○	○	○
In international organizations	○	○	○	○
In nongovernmental organizations	○	○	○	○
In the media	○	○	○	○

21. How satisfied are you with the following aspects of the fellowship?

	Not at all satisfied (1)	2	3	4	Extremely satisfied (5)
Stipend	○	○	○	○	○
Benefits	○	○	○	○	○
Support from fellowship staff	○	○	○	○	○
Resources provided by USIP (space, computer, etc.)	○	○	○	○	○
Support to conduct research outside of Washington, DC	○	○	○	○	○
Research assistant	○	○	○	○	○
Opportunities to interact with other Fellows	○	○	○	○	○
Opportunities to interact with USIP staff	○	○	○	○	○
Opportunities to participate in USIP events	○	○	○	○	○

22. Have you recommended the fellowship to others?

○ Yes
○ No
○ Can't recall

23. Would you recommend the fellowship to others?

○ Yes
○ No
○ Don't know

If not, please tell us why

24. Is there anything else that you would like to tell the committee about the senior fellows program?

Appendix C
Survey of Peace and Security Experts

1. Brief survey of peace and security fellowships

The National Academy of Sciences is conducting an assessment of peace and security fellowships. We are contacting individuals in academia, government, and nongovernmental organizations to ask a few questions about their opinions regarding the impact of these fellowships.

All answers are anonymous and confidential. We do not ask for nor record your name or affiliation. Your answers will only be reported in the aggregate, and will never be reported in a way that can be linked back to you.

This information will be collected and published in a report, which will be available on the National Academies Press website (www.nap.edu) at the project's completion (tentatively the end of August 2008).

1. On a scale from 1 to 5 where 5 is extremly familiar and 1 is not at all familiar, how familiar are you with the Woodrow Wilson International Center for Scholars fellowship program?

  ◯ 1 (Not at all familiar)
  ◯ 2
  ◯ 3
  ◯ 4
  ◯ 5 (Extremely familiar)

2. On a scale from 1 to 5 where 5 is extremly familiar and 1 is not at all familiar, how familiar are you with the U.S. Department of State Franklin fellowships program?

  ◯ 1 (Not at all familiar)
  ◯ 2
  ◯ 3
  ◯ 4
  ◯ 5 (Extremely familiar)

3. On a scale from 1 to 5 where 5 is extremly familiar and 1 is not at all familiar, how familiar are you with the AAAS Science & Technology Policy Fellowships in National Defense & Global Security?

  ◯ 1 (Not at all familiar)
  ◯ 2
  ◯ 3
  ◯ 4
  ◯ 5 (Extremely familiar)

4. On a scale from 1 to 5 where 5 is extremly familiar and 1 is not at all familiar, how familiar are you with the U.S. Institute of Peace Jennings Randolph Senior Fellowships?

◯ 1 (Not at all familiar)
◯ 2
◯ 3
◯ 4
◯ 5 (Extremely familiar)

2. Page 2 of 4

1. Overall how prestigious do you think each program is? Please use a scale from 1 to 5, where 1 is not at all prestigious and 5 is extremely prestigious.

	1 (Not at all prestigious)	2	3	4	5 (Extremely prestigious)	Unsure
Woodrow Wilson International Center for Scholars fellowships	○	○	○	○	○	○
U.S. Department of State Franklin fellowships	○	○	○	○	○	○
AAAS Science & Technology Policy Fellowships in National Defense & Global Security	○	○	○	○	○	○
U.S. Institute of Peace Jennings Randolph Senior Fellowships	○	○	○	○	○	○

3. Page 3 of 4

Now we would like to conclude the survey by asking you a few questions just about the U.S. Institute of Peace Jennings Randolph Senior Fellowship Program

1. Have you known any U.S. Institute of Peace Jennings Randolph Senior Fellows?

○ Yes
○ No
○ Unsure

2. On a scale from 1 to 5 where 1 is not at all important and 5 is extremely important, how important do you think the Jennings Randolph Senior Fellowships are

	1 (Not at all important)	2	3	4	5 (Extremely important)	Unsure
in providing opportunities to bring people to Washington to network with experts in peace and security issues?	○	○	○	○	○	○
to increasing knowledge on peace and security topics, such as the nature of conflict or conflict resolution?	○	○	○	○	○	○
to developing new tools to manage, mitigate, or resolve conflicts?	○	○	○	○	○	○

3. On a scale from 1 to 5, where 1 is not at all and 5 is to a very great extent, would you say that the Jennings Randolph Senior Fellows

	1 (Not at all)	2	3	4	5 (To a very Great Extent)	Unsure
perform cutting-edge research?	○	○	○	○	○	○
support policy-makers by providing analyses, policy options, or advice?	○	○	○	○	○	○

4. On a scale from 1 to 5, where 1 is not at all and 5 is to a very great extent, would you say that the return on investment that the U.S. Institute of Peace receives from the Jennings Randolph Senior Fellowship program is well worth the cost?

○ 1 (Not at all)
○ 2
○ 3
○ 4
○ 5 (To a very great extent)
○ Unsure

5. Have you ever recommended anyone apply to the fellowship program?

○ Yes

○ No

○ Unsure

6. Is there anything else you would like to tell us about the fellowship program?

4. Page 4 of 4

1. My employment position is best described as being in...

○ Academia (including research centers and institutes)

○ Government

○ Nongovernmental organization

Appendix D
Top Foreign Policy Problems Identified by Chicago Council on Foreign Relations Interviews with Foreign Policy Leaders, 1986–2002

Table D-1 Top foreign policy problems identified in 1986

Issue	Percent	Fellows after
Russia/dealings with Russia	46	
Arms Control (Nuclear weapons, too much military equipment sold or given to other countries)	33	
Latin/South/Central America	28	
Balance of Payments (Trade deficit, too much money going out of country, import of foreign products)	17	
Mid-East Situation (Non-specific)	15	
Terrorism	11	
Third World Problems (Poverty, underdevelopment)	11	
International Trade (Free trade with all countries, some countries too strict with trade policies)	9	
World Economy	8	
Stronger Foreign Policy Needed (U.S. is compromising)	8	
South Africa/Apartheid	8	
War (Threat of war, threat of nuclear war)	6	
Keeping Peace (Should have better relations)	5	
Dealing with Communism	4	
Devaluation of the Dollar/Money	3	
Too Much Military Involvement in Other Countries	3	
Changing Relations with African Countries	2	
Foreign Aid (Too much sent to other countries)	2	
Immigration (Illegal aliens)	2	
Domestic Problems (Crime, unemployment, government waste, etc.)	2	
Human Rights Campaign	2	
China/Relations with China/China Economy	1	

Issue	Count
Oil Problems (Oil shortage, dependency on oil-producing countries)	1
Cuba	1
Our Relationship with Japan	1
Our Relationship with Israel	0.5
Drugs (Smuggling, coming from other countries)	0.5

Table D-2 Top foreign policy problems identified in 1990

Issue	Fellows before	Percent	Fellows after
Iraq (Saddam Hussein)		44	
Mid-East Situation (Non-specific)		29	
Russia/dealings with Russia		21	
International Trade (Free trade with all countries, some countries too strict with trade policies)		18	
World Economy		14	
Keeping Peace (Should have better relations)		13	
Impact of Freedom in Eastern Europe		12	
Our Relationship with Japan		9	
Third World Problems (Poverty, underdevelopment)		8	
Stronger Foreign Policy Needed (U.S. is compromising)		7	
The Economic Unification of Europe		7	
Arms Control (Nuclear weapons, too much military equipment sold or given to other countries)		6	
Environment (environmental policies, oil spills, energy sources)		6	
Latin/South/Central America		6	
Balance of Payments (Trade deficit, too much money going out of country, import of foreign products)		5	
Weak leadership (honesty in government/double standards with other countries)		5	
Our Relationship with Israel		4	
Too Much Military Involvement in Other Countries		4	
China/Relations with China/China Economy		3	
Oil Problems (Oil shortage, dependency on oil-producing countries)		3	

Issue	Count
War (Threat of war, threat of nuclear war)	3
Don't Understand Foreign Culture	3
Foreign Aid (Too much sent to other countries)	2
Domestic Problems (Crime, unemployment, government waste, etc.)	2
Human Rights Campaign	2
Drugs (Smuggling, coming from other countries)	2
Dealing with Communism	2
Terrorism	1
Changing Relations with African Countries	1
Immigration (Illegal aliens)	1
Devaluation of the Dollar/Money	1
Cuba	0.5
South Africa/Apartheid	0.5

Table D-3 Top foreign policy problems identified in 1994

Issue	Fellows before	Percent	Fellows after
International Trade (Free trade with all countries, some countries too strict with trade policies)		24	
Russia/dealings with Russia		23	
Weak leadership (honesty in government/double standards with other countries)		19	
Stronger Foreign Policy Needed (U.S. is compromising)		16	
Our Relationship with Bosnia		16	
Arms Control (Nuclear weapons, too much military equipment sold or given to other countries)		14	
World Economy		11	
Mid-East Situation (Non-specific)		7	
Keeping Peace (Should have better relations)		7	
U.S. Role as World Leader/World's Police		6	
Third World Problems (Poverty, underdevelopment)		5	
China/Relations with China/China Economy		5	
Foreign Aid (Too much sent to other countries)		5	

Environment (environmental policies, oil spills, energy sources)	4
Our Relationship with North Korea	4
Our Relationship with Israel	3
Immigration (Illegal aliens)	3
Our Relationship with Japan	3
Balance of Payments (Trade deficit, too much money going out of country, import of foreign products)	2
War (Threat of war, threat of nuclear war)	2
Don't Understand Foreign Culture	2
Domestic Problems (Crime, unemployment, government waste, etc.)	2
United Nations (relations with UN, UN not doing its job)	2
Human Rights Campaign	2
Too Much Military Involvement in Other Countries	2
Dealing with Communism	2
South Africa/Apartheid	2
Terrorism	1
Iraq (Saddam Hussein)	1
Foreign Relations	1
Changing Relations with African Countries	1
Jobs going overseas (Keep our jobs in U.S.)	1
Latin/South/Central America	1
Cuba	1
Impact of Freedom in Eastern Europe	1
Overpopulation	1
Countries taking advantage of us	1

Table D-4 Top foreign policy problems identified in 1998

Issue	Fellows before	Percent	Fellows after
World Economy		21	
Iraq (Saddam Hussein)		18	
Arms Control (Nuclear weapons, too much military equipment sold or given to other countries)		15	
Russia/dealings with Russia		13	
Japan/Asian Economy/Crisis		13	
Mid-East Situation (Non-specific)		12	
Terrorism		10	
China/Relations with China/China Economy		9	
U.S. Role as World Leader/World's Police		8	
Stronger Foreign Policy Needed (U.S. is compromising)		6	
International Trade (Free trade with all countries, some countries too strict with trade policies)		6	
Keeping Peace (Should have better relations)		6	
Third World Problems (Poverty, underdevelopment)		4	
Foreign Relations		4	
Our Relationship with North Korea		3	
Our Relationship with Bosnia		3	
Countries taking advantage of us		3	
Trade (non-specific)		2	
Religious issues/Fanaticism		2	
Our Relationship with Israel		2	
Environment (environmental policies, oil spills, energy sources)		2	
Balance of Payments (Trade deficit, too much money going out of country, import of foreign products)		2	
Jobs going overseas (Keep our jobs in U.S.)		2	
Weak leadership (honesty in government/double standards with other countries)		2	
Unrest in Israel/Israel and Palestine		1	
Changing Relations with African Countries		1	
Immigration (Illegal aliens)		1	

World Peace	1
National Security	1
Oil Problems (Oil shortage, dependency on oil-producing countries)	1
Domestic Problems (Crime, unemployment, government waste, etc.)	1
Latin/South/Central America	1
Devaluation of the Dollar/Money	1
United Nations (relations with UN, UN not doing its job)	1
Human Rights Campaign	1
Drugs (Smuggling, coming from other countries)	1
Cuba	1
Overpopulation	1
The Economic Unification of Europe	1
Our Relationship with Japan	1
Instability of foreign markets	1
Politics	1
Kosovo	1
Foreign Aid (Too much sent to other countries)	0.5
War (Threat of war, threat of nuclear war)	0.5
Don't Understand Foreign Culture	0.5
Too Much Military Involvement in Other Countries	0.5
Dealing with Communism	0.5
We need to help the children (Needy children/children of foreign countries)	0.5
Impact of Freedom in Eastern Europe	0.5
Hostages	0.5
South Africa/Apartheid	0.5
Need to Help the Needy (Non-specific)	0.5

Table D-5 Top foreign policy problems identified in 2002

Issue	Fellows before	Percent	Fellows after
Terrorism		50	
Mid-East Situation (Non-specific)		38	
Unrest in Israel/Israel and Palestine		16	
India and Pakistan issues		14	
Arms Control (Nuclear weapons, too much military equipment sold or given to other countries)		9	
Third World Problems (Poverty, underdevelopment)		8	
World Economy		7	
Stronger Foreign Policy Needed (U.S. is compromising)		7	
China/Relations with China/China Economy		6	
International Trade (Free trade with all countries, some countries too strict with trade policies)		5	
Trade (non-specific)		5	
Re-defining America's Role in an unstable environment		4	
Iraq (Saddam Hussein)		4	
Foreign Relations		4	
Changing Relations with African Countries		4	
Religious issues/Fanaticism		4	
Foreign Aid (Too much sent to other countries)		3	
Situation in Afghanistan		3	
Loss of respect for U.S. abroad		3	
Relations with Europe		3	
AIDS/virus/disease/world sickness		3	
Our Relationship with Israel		2	
Environment (environmental policies, oil spills, energy sources)		2	
Balance of Payments (Trade deficit, too much money going out of country, import of foreign products)		2	
Russia/dealings with Russia		2	
Immigration (Illegal aliens)		2	
World Peace		2	
National Security		2	
Oil Problems (Oil shortage, dependency on oil-producing countries)		2	

War (Threat of war, threat of nuclear war)	2
Don't Understand Foreign Culture	2
Stay out of the affairs of other countries	2
Gap between rich and poor nations	2
Relations with far East countries	2
Globalization (non-specific)	2
U.S. Role as World Leader/World's Police	1
Domestic Problems (Crime, unemployment, government waste, etc.)	1
Jobs going overseas (Keep our jobs in U.S.)	1
Latin/South/Central America	1
Weak leadership (honesty in government/double standards with other countries)	1
Devaluation of the Dollar/Money	1
United Nations (relations with UN, UN not doing its job)	1
Human Rights Campaign	1
Too Much Military Involvement in Other Countries	1
Industrial competitiveness/economically or technically behind/declining productivity	1
U.S. relationship with NATO countries	1
Lack of trust/trust between countries	1
Drugs (Smuggling, coming from other countries)	1
bin Laden	1
Dealing with Communism	0.5
We need to help the children (Needy children/children of foreign countries)	0.5
Cuba	0.5